Rheumatology Pearls for the Primary Care Physician

Editor

BRIAN F. MANDELL

RHEUMATIC DISEASE CLINICS OF NORTH AMERICA

www.rheumatic.theclinics.com

Consulting Editor
MICHAEL H. WEISMAN

May 2022 • Volume 48 • Number 2

ELSEVIER

1600 John F. Kennedy Boulevard • Suite 1800 • Philadelphia, Pennsylvania, 19103-2899
http://www.theclinics.com

RHEUMATIC DISEASE CLINICS OF NORTH AMERICA Volume 48, Number 2
May 2022 ISSN 0889-857X, ISBN 13: 978-0-323-93919-5

Editor: Joanna Collett
Developmental Editor: Karen Solomon

Rheumatic Disease Clinics of North America (ISSN 0889-857X) is published quarterly by Elsevier Inc., 360 Park Avenue South, New York, NY 10010-1710. Months of issue are February, May, August, and November. Business and editorial offices: 1600 John F. Kennedy Boulevard, Suite 1800, Philadelphia, PA 19103-2899. Periodicals postage paid at New York, NY and additional mailing offices. Subscription prices are USD 366.00 per year for US individuals, USD 1020.00 per year for US institutions, USD 100.00 per year for US students and residents, USD 431.00 per year for Canadian individuals, USD 1040.00 per year for Canadian institutions, USD 100.00 per year for Canadian students/residents, USD 470.00 per year for international individuals, USD 1040.00 per year for international institutions, and USD 230.00 per year for foreign students/residents. To receive student/ resident rate, orders must be accompanied by name of affiliated institution, date of term, and the *signature* of program/residency coordinator on institution letterhead. Orders will be billed at individual rate until proof of status received. Foreign air speed delivery is included in all *Clinics* subscription prices. All prices are subject to change without notice. **POSTMASTER:** Send address changes to *Rheumatic Disease Clinics of North America,* Elsevier Health Sciences Division, Subscription Customer Service, 3251 Riverport Lane, Maryland Heights, MO 63043. **Customer Service: 1-800-654-2452 (US and Canada). From outside of the US and Canada: 314-447-8871. Fax: 314-447-8029. For print support, e-mail: JournalsCustomerService-usa@elsevier.com. For online support, e-mail: JournalsOnlineSupport-usa@elsevier.com.**

Reprints. For copies of 100 or more of articles in this publication, please contact the Commercial Reprints Department, Elsevier Inc., 360 Park Avenue South, New York, New York, 10010-1710; Tel.: +1-212-633-3874, Fax: +1-212-633-3820, and E-mail: reprints@elsevier.com.

Rheumatic Disease Clinics of North America is covered in *MEDLINE/PubMed (Index Medicus), Current Contents/Clinical Medicine, Science Citation Index, ISI/BIOMED,* and *EMBASE/Excerpta Medica.*

Contributors

CONSULTING EDITOR

MICHAEL H. WEISMAN, MD
Adjunct Professor of Medicine, Stanford University, Distinguished Professor of Medicine, Emeritus, David Geffen School of Medicine at UCLA, Professor of Medicine Emeritus, Cedars-Sinai Medical Center, Los Angeles, California, USA

EDITOR

BRIAN F. MANDELL, MD, PhD, MACR, MACP
Professor and Chairman Department of Academic Medicine, Department Rheumatologic and Immunologic Diseases, Cleveland Clinic Lerner College of Medicine, at Case Western Reserve University, Cleveland Clinic, Cleveland, Ohio, USA

AUTHORS

ANNE R. BASS, MD
Professor of Clinical Medicine, Hospital for Special Surgery, Weill Cornell Medicine, New York, New York, USA

BONNIE L. BERMAS, MD
UT Southwestern Medical Center, Dallas, Texas, USA

JOEL A. BLOCK, MD
The Willard L Wood MD Professor, and Director, Division of Rheumatology, Rush University Medical Center, Chicago, Illinois, USA

CASSANDRA CALABRESE, DO
Associate Staff, Department of Rheumatologic and Immunologic Disease, Department of Infectious Disease, Cleveland Clinic Foundation, Cleveland, Ohio, USA

ADELA CASTRO-GUTIERREZ, MD
UT Southwestern Medical Center, Dallas, Texas, USA

DMITRIY CHERNY, MD
Fellow, Division of Rheumatology, Rush University Medical Center, Chicago, Illinois, USA

JOHN J. CUSH, MD
Professor of Internal Medicine, Rheumatic Disease Division, The University of Texas Southwestern Medical School, Dallas, Texas, USA

SARAH EL CHAMI, MBBS
Rheumatology Fellow, The University of Kansas Health System, Kansas City, Kansas, USA

LYN D. FERGUSON, MBChB (Hons), PhD, MRCP(UK)
Institute of Cardiovascular and Medical Sciences, University of Glasgow, Glasgow, United Kingdom

NILASHA GHOSH, MD
Hospital for Special Surgery, Weill Cornell Medicine, New York, New York, USA

SUSAN M. GOODMAN, MD
Attending Rheumatologist, Hospital for Special Surgery, Professor of Clinical Medicine, Weill Cornell Medicine, New York, New York, USA

CARMEN E. GOTA, MD
Staff Rheumatologist, Assistant Professor of Medicine, Case Western Reserve Cleveland Clinic School of Medicine, Cleveland, Ohio, USA

SARAH F. KELLER, MD, MA
Department of Rheumatic & Immunologic Diseases, Staff Rheumatologist, The Cleveland Clinic, Cleveland, Ohio, USA

ANDREW L. MAMMEN, MD, PhD
Muscle Disease Unit, Laboratory of Muscle Stem Cells and Gene Regulation, National Institute of Arthritis and Musculoskeletal and Skin Diseases, National Institutes of Health, Departments of Neurology and Medicine, Johns Hopkins University School of Medicine, Baltimore, Maryland, USA

BRIAN F. MANDELL, MD, PhD, MACP, FACR
Professor and Chairman Department of Academic Medicine, Professor and Chairman of Academic Medicine, Department of Rheumatic & Immunologic Diseases, The Cleveland Clinic, Cleveland, Ohio, USA

IAIN B. MCINNES, MBChB, PhD, FRCP
Professor, Institute of Infection, Immunity and Inflammation, University of Glasgow, Glasgow, United Kingdom

PHILIP J. MEASE, MD, MACR
Director, Rheumatology Research, Swedish Medical Center/Providence St. Joseph Health, Clinical Professor, University of Washington School of Medicine, Seattle, Washington, USA

RAND A. NASHI, MD
Clinical Fellow, Division of Rheumatology, Beth Israel Deaconess Medical Center, Boston, Massachusetts, USA

NAVEED SATTAR, MBChB, PhD, FRCP
Professor, Institute of Cardiovascular and Medical Sciences, University of Glasgow, Glasgow, United Kingdom

ROBERT H. SHMERLING, MD
Associate Physician, Division of Rheumatology, Beth Israel Deaconess Medical Center, Senior Editor, Harvard Health Publications, Harvard Medical School, Corresponding Faculty, Harvard Medical School, Boston, Massachusetts, USA

JASON M. SPRINGER, MD, MS
Assistant Professor, Vanderbilt University Medical Center, Nashville, TN, USA

KRISTEN YOUNG, MD
UT Southwestern Medical Center, Dallas, Texas, USA

DIANE ZISA, MD
Rheumatology Fellow, Hospital for Special Surgery, New York, New York, USA

Contents

Foreword: Rheumatology Pearls for the Primary Care Physician   xi

Michael H. Weisman

Preface: It Takes Oysters to Generate Pearls   xiii

Brian F. Mandell

Vaccinations in Patients with Rheumatic Disease: Consider Disease and Therapy   397

Cassandra Calabrese

> Patients with rheumatic diseases are susceptible to infections due to their underlying disease states as well as from immunosuppressive medications, highlighting the importance of vaccination, these same factors also pose challenges to vaccine efficacy, safety, and uptake. This article reviews the impact of immunosuppressive therapies and rheumatic disease on vaccine efficacy in this vulnerable patient population as well as discusses best practices.

Rheumatic Complications of Immune Checkpoint Inhibitors   411

Nilasha Ghosh and Anne R. Bass

> Immune checkpoint inhibitors activate the immune system to combat cancer. In doing so, however, they can cause immune-related adverse events (irAEs), including rheumatic syndromes, such as inflammatory arthritis, polymyalgia rheumatica, and myositis. This article reviews rheumatic irAEs that may be encountered in the general medicine practice and provides guidance to support prompt recognition, referral, and treatment of these patients.

Managing Cardiovascular Risk in Patients with Rheumatic Disease   429

Lyn D. Ferguson, Naveed Sattar, and Iain B. McInnes

> Individuals with rheumatoid arthritis, systemic lupus erythematosus, or gout have increased risk of cardiovascular disease (CVD) compared with the general population. This risk relates to a combination of traditional cardiovascular risk factors and disease-specific factors. Screening for CVD is important because CVD contributes to significant morbidity and mortality. Management includes tight control of disease activity to reduce inflammation, but with care to minimize use of nonsteroidal anti-inflammatory drugs and prolonged courses of high-dose corticosteroids. Traditional cardiovascular risk factors should be managed with a combination of lifestyle interventions and pharmacotherapy. The decision to start antihypertensive and lipid-lowering therapy should be based on individual CVD risk.

Statin-Associated Myalgias and Muscle Injury—Recognizing and Managing Both While Still Lowering the Low-Density Lipoprotein   445

Andrew L. Mammen

Although statins are generally safe and well tolerated, some patients experience muscle complaints that can be attributed to their use. Those with muscle discomfort but no demonstrable muscle weakness or creatine kinase (CK) elevations may have statin-associated muscle symptoms. Individuals with elevated CK levels, with or without muscle discomfort or weakness, may have statin-associated myotoxicity. Rare patients have statin-associated autoimmune myopathy, a disease characterized by proximal muscle weakness, elevated CK levels, and autoantibodies recognizing hydroxy-methyl-glutaryl coenzyme A reductase. In this review, the author provides the clinician with a practical approach to diagnosing and managing patients with each of these statin side effects.

Perioperative Management of Rheumatic Disease and Therapies   455

Diane Zisa and Susan M. Goodman

Patients with rheumatic disease, including those with systemic lupus erythematous, rheumatoid arthritis, and spondyloarthritis, use total hip and knee arthroplasties at high rates. They represent a particularly vulnerable population in the perioperative setting because of their diseases and the immunosuppressant therapies used to treat them. Careful planning among internists, medical specialists, and the surgical team must therefore occur preoperatively to minimize risks in the postoperative period, particularly infection. Management of immunosuppressant medications, such as conventional synthetic disease-modifying antirheumatic drugs and targeted therapies including biologics, is one avenue by which this infectious risk can be mitigated.

Fibromyalgia: Recognition and Management in the Primary Care Office   467

Carmen E. Gota

Fibromyalgia is a chronic pain condition manifested by chronic generalized pain, fatigue, disordered sleep, and cognitive difficulties, persistent for at least 3 months. Other common complaints/conditions include symptoms of irritable bowel syndrome, headaches, intermittent paresthesias, and various mood disorders. Women are more commonly affected than men. The treatment approach should be individualized and focused on associated mood disorders, sleep, exercise, correction of maladaptive responses to pain, and coping with stress.

Management and Cure of Gouty Arthritis   479

Sarah F. Keller and Brian F. Mandell

Gout is the most common inflammatory arthritis in the United States. Gouty arthritis is associated with significant morbidity and mortality and is the result of chronic hyperuricemia. Gout is effectively managed and potentially cured by decreasing the overall urate burden with serum urate–lowering therapy. When serum urate is maintained at less than 6.0 mg/dL, urate deposition is resolved, and gout can be cured. Unfortunately, because of less than optimal physician monitoring and dose escalation, many patients do not achieve these urate levels.

Update on the Treatment of Giant Cell Arteritis and Polymyalgia Rheumatica   493

Sarah El Chami and Jason M. Springer

Giant cell arteritis (GCA) and polymyalgia rheumatica (PMR) are considered 2 diseases on the same spectrum due to their many underlying similarities. In recent years, both diseases have witnessed both diagnostic and treatment advances, which shaped the way we manage them. In this article, the authors focus on different diagnostic modalities in GCA as well as the presence of different clinical phenotypes and the role of screening for aortic involvement. The authors also discuss traditional treatments and the role of evolving steroid-sparing agents in the management of both GCA and PMR.

Suspecting and Diagnosing the Patient with Spondyloarthritis and What to Expect from Therapy   507

Philip J. Mease

Spondyloarthritis is a common rheumatologic disease, present in up to 2% of the population, characterized by inflammatory arthritis, often with enthesitis, dactylitis, spondylitis, and skin disease. It has historically been characterized as ankylosing spondylitis, psoriatic arthritis, arthritis associated with inflammatory bowel disease, reactive arthritis, and undifferentiated spondyloarthritis. These subsets are now classified as axial-predominant and peripheral-predominant spondyloarthritis. This article provides an updated understanding of disease classification and practical advice about diagnosis to aid in the determination of which patients should be referred to rheumatology. It is important to provide patients the opportunity to have early and effective therapy.

Pregnancy and Management in Women with Rheumatoid Arthritis, Systemic Lupus Erythematosus, and Obstetric Antiphospholipid Syndrome   523

Adela Castro-Gutierrez, Kristen Young, and Bonnie L. Bermas

Management of women with rheumatoid arthritis (RA), systemic lupus erythematosus (SLE), and obstetric antiphospholipid syndrome (APS) during pregnancy presents unique clinical challenges. Women with both RA and SLE can have disease flares during pregnancy, leading to pregnancy complications, such as preeclampsia, small-for-gestational-age infants, and preterm delivery. Disease should be under control prior to conception. Women with obstetric APS need to be anticoagulated during pregnancy. Many but not all antirheumatic medications can be used during pregnancy and lactation.

Rheumatoid Arthritis: Early Diagnosis and Treatment   537

John J. Cush

Rheumatoid arthritis (RA) is a chronic, progressive inflammatory disorder that manifests as a symmetric polyarthritis of small and large joints that may lead to joint and periarticular structural damage and the consequences of systemic inflammation. This overview of early RA examines the unmet needs and challenges in RA, how to best diagnose RA, and pitfalls in early diagnosis and treatment. The rules for referral to a rheumatologist are reviewed. Primary care physicians are at the front line of early diagnosis and need to start disease-modifying therapy as soon as a diagnosis of RA is established.

Management of Knee Osteoarthritis: What Internists Need to Know   **549**

Joel A. Block and Dmitriy Cherny

Knee osteoarthritis (OA) is a common and morbid condition. No disease-modifying therapies exist; hence the goals of current treatment are to palliate pain and to retain function. OA pain is significantly influenced by the placebo effect. Nonpharmacologic interventions are essential and have been shown to improve outcomes. Canes, unloading braces, and therapeutic heating/cooling may be valuable. Pharmacotherapy options include topical and oral nonsteroidal anti-inflammatory drugs, duloxetine, and periodic intra-articular glucocorticoids and hyaluronans. Opioids, intra-articular stem cells, and platelet-rich plasma are not recommended. Novel targets such as nerve growth factor are under investigation and may be approved soon for OA pain.

Antinuclear Antibody Testing for the Diagnosis of Systemic Lupus Erythematosus   **569**

Rand A. Nashi and Robert H. Shmerling

Systemic lupus erythematosus (SLE) is an autoimmune inflammatory condition that may involve multiple organ systems. Although the antinuclear antibody (ANA) test is positive in nearly every case of SLE, it is not specific for this disease and must be interpreted in the appropriate clinical context. Key features that warrant ANA testing include unexplained multisystem inflammatory disease, symmetric joint pain with inflammatory features, photosensitive rash, and cytopenias. ANA staining patterns and more specific autoantibody testing may be helpful in diagnosis of suspected SLE or ANA-associated disease. For patients with nonspecific symptoms, such as malaise and fatigue, ANA testing is of limited value.

RHEUMATIC DISEASE CLINICS OF NORTH AMERICA

FORTHCOMING ISSUES

August 2022
Treatment Guideline Development and Implementation
Michael Ward, *Editor*

November 2022
Environmental Triggers for Rheumatic Diseases
Bryant R. England, *Editor*

February 2023
Cardiovascular Complications of Chronic Rheumatic Diseases
Elaine Husni and George A. Karpouzas, *Editors*

RECENT ISSUES

February 2022
Pediatric Rheumatology Comes of Age: Part II
Yukiko Kimura and Laura E. Schanberg, *Editors*

November 2021
Pediatric Rheumatology Comes of Age: Part I
Yukiko Kimura and Laura E. Schanberg, *Editors*

August 2021
Lupus
Alfred H.J. Kim and Zahi Touma, *Editors*

THE CLINICS ARE AVAILABLE ONLINE!
Access your subscription at:
www.theclinics.com

Foreword

Rheumatology Pearls for the Primary Care Physician

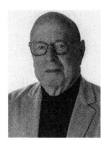

Michael H. Weisman, MD
Consulting Editor

Brian Mandell has done a masterful job in assembling topics for the primary care physician that correspond to his experience with words of wisdom, called "pearls." He has provided summaries from extremely knowledgeable specialists that reflect on their clinical experiences, their tough-minded view of the literature, and most importantly, what is not in the literature or in guidelines. He talks about the time it takes for pearls to develop, using the analogy about their generation to point out that decision making by experts is something that is based on how we integrate each experience into the next. It is similar to what I have always told Fellow applicants about what they face in the next 2 years: that is, the first year they learn the rules; the second year, they learn that the rules really don't apply to the next patient. It is that jump, or leap, into the world where the rules don't work, guidelines are insufficient, and the literature is biased; that is where critical thinking must take place. We are very appreciative of this issue, which gives us a peek into how our experienced clinicians make a diagnosis and institute therapy.

Michael H. Weisman, MD
10800 Wilshire Blvd. #404
Los Angeles, CA 90024, USA

E-mail address:
michael.weisman@cshs.org

Rheum Dis Clin N Am 48 (2022) xi
https://doi.org/10.1016/j.rdc.2022.03.003
0889-857X/22/© 2022 Published by Elsevier Inc.

Preface

It Takes Oysters to Generate Pearls

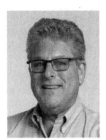

Brian F. Mandell, MD, PhD, MACR, MACP
Editor

For this issue of *Rheumatic Disease Clinics of North America*, "Rheumatology pearls for the primary care physician," I have asked a selected group of experienced clinicians with special interests to provide their personal overviews of specific clinical topics. I asked them to direct their comments to seasoned clinicians who do not share the author's more specific experiences.

The internal medicine subspecialty of rheumatology encompasses a broad range of clinical disorders spanning the gamut from regional musculoskeletal pain syndromes to complex systemic autoimmune and inflammatory conditions associated with severe morbidity and mortality. These may be triggered (or their expression modified) by exogenous factors, genetic background, or immune dysregulation that has occurred from known or idiopathic reasons. Specific rheumatic disorders occur with various frequency. Some are relatively uncommon but threaten patients' quality of life to a degree that early recognition is mandatory. And there lies a major challenge, particularly for clinicians responsible for delivering primary care: how to recognize, initially manage, and appropriately refer patients with disorders that can be life threatening. These are disorders that the clinician may not be totally comfortable making the diagnosis, yet knowing that there is likely to be a significant delay in the ability to have their patient seen by an appropriate subspecialist. Complicating the decision process is the fact that many of these rheumatic diseases can at least superficially mimic each other in their initial presentation.

Perhaps based on recall from a few lectures or rotations in medical school, or perhaps drawing from observed behaviors without detailed explanation from subspecialist consultants, there is a widespread reliance on the use of serologic immunologic testing to make a diagnosis or dictate therapy and referral. But most "autoimmune" serologic tests are rarely definitive, and their use is far more valuable in supporting or occasionally refuting a potential diagnosis that has been suggested by careful review of the patients' history and physical examination. Unexplained fatigue accompanied by chronic diffuse pain, tingling, or subjective numbness and "brain fog" does not equate with having an autoimmune etiology, even if the ANA or SSA serologic test is positive.

Some general health management decisions that need to be made when caring for patients already diagnosed with rheumatic or immunologic diseases warrant specific information or experience: appropriate management decisions, even commonly occurring ones like vaccination or lipid management, may differ from those made for other patients. This can be especially challenging for the busy clinician for whom these patients represent a very small percentage of their practice. And thus enters the oyster in the title of this preface.

The value of pearls in the real world stems in large part from the recognition that they take time to develop, and that they don't develop everywhere. Just as all oysters don't generate pearls, it takes time and environment, and it is not reasonable to think that all clinicians, even very experienced ones, can realistically have the same exposure to the patients discussed in this volume OR have the time to search the literature to glean guidance for decision making when they are encountered in clinic (and it is a leap of faith to think that the literature always provides adequate *evidence* to appropriately guide that decision process).

I am hoping that the brief summaries provided in this issue will provide readers, primary care clinicians as well as subspecialists with clinical pearls generated from the appropriate clinicians to assist in the management of our patients with rheumatic disorders. I've asked the authors to be pragmatic more than theoretic in providing their insights. And I've encouraged them to extend their comments beyond the published literature when that literature is insufficient to enable decision making, drawing on the time that they have personally spent reading about and providing hands-on care for their patients.

Brian F. Mandell, MD, PhD, MACR, MACP
Department Rheumatologic and
Immunologic Diseases
Cleveland Clinic Lerner College of Medicine
at Case Western Reserve University
Cleveland Clinic
9500 Euclid Avenue A50
Cleveland, OH 44195, USA

E-mail address:
mandelb@ccf.org

Vaccinations in Patients with Rheumatic Disease
Consider Disease and Therapy

Cassandra Calabrese, DO

KEYWORDS

- Rheumatic diseases • Immunosuppression • Vaccine • Immunogenicity • Biologics
- DMARD • Infection

KEY POINTS

- Influenza vaccine immunogenicity is reduced by rituximab and methotrexate.
- Pneumococcal vaccine immunogenicity is reduced by rituximab, methotrexate, and possibly abatacept and tofacitinib.
- When possible, for patients receiving treatment with rituximab, administration of influenza and pneumococcal vaccines should be administered 6 months after and 4 weeks prior to the next rituximab dose to maximize immunogenicity.
- Live vaccines are contraindicated in the setting of biologic therapy but can be considered in the setting of lower-dose immunosuppression.
- The recombinant herpes zoster vaccine has not been heavily studied in patients with rheumatic diseases; however, it should be recommended with informed decision making.

INTRODUCTION

Risk of infection is increased in patients with rheumatic diseases secondary to both their underlying disease states as well as from immunosuppressive medications used for their treatment. There are many unique aspects of vaccinology in rheumatology patients, including the particular infectious morbidity in this patient population, and perhaps most importantly the impact of conventional synthetic and biologic disease-modifying antirheumatic drugs (DMARDs) on vaccine safety and efficacy. The introduction of biologic therapies has revolutionized the treatment of rheumatic diseases, yet accompanying this is a further increased risk of infection, highlighting the importance of vaccines even further. When considering vaccinating rheumatic diseases patients, disease activity, type of immunosuppression, and timing of vaccine

This article originally appeared in the Medical Clinics of North America, Volume 105, Issue 2, March 2021.

Department of Rheumatologic & Immunologic Disease, Cleveland Clinic Foundation, 9500 Euclid Avenue, Desk A50, Cleveland, OH 44195, USA

E-mail address: calabrc@ccf.org

Twitter: @CCalabreseDO (C.C.)

Rheum Dis Clin N Am 48 (2022) 397–409
https://doi.org/10.1016/j.rdc.2022.02.001
0889-857X/22/© 2022 Elsevier Inc. All rights reserved.

administration must be considered to optimize both efficacy and safety. Although it is mainly the rheumatologist's role to keep up to date with vaccine administration and recommendations, awareness and communication with other specialists as well as primary care providers and internists are key, because ultimately it is a group effort. Although it is well-known that vaccines are the best mode of infection prevention, their uptake remains low in patients with rheumatic diseases. The objective of this review is to summarize the impact of immunosuppressive therapies and rheumatic disease on vaccine efficacy in this unique patient population and to present best practices.

GENERAL PRINCIPLES AND RECOMMENDATIONS

The recommended adult immunization schedule is updated annually by the Advisory Committee on Immunization Practices (ACIP) and includes recommendations for immunizing against more than 10 vaccine-preventable infections. The recommendations are stratified by patient population, and under each vaccine recommendation are bullet point recommendations for special situations, which include immunocompromising conditions, for example, patients with rheumatic diseases receiving immunosuppression. The major rheumatology societies have released guidelines as well, some of which are outdated and are discussed later, with the 3 most important vaccines to consider in patients with rheumatic diseases highlighted: influenza, the pneumococcal series, and herpes zoster (HZ).

Vaccination Against Influenza

The American College of Rheumatology (ACR) has published immunization recommendations for patients with rheumatoid arthritis (RA) only and supports universal immunization against seasonal influenza,[1] whereas the European League Against Rheumatism (EULAR) recommendations encourage influenza vaccination be considered for the majority of patients with rheumatic diseases,[2] which is reflective of differing immunization practices between the United States and European countries.

Seasonal influenza vaccine should be administered to all rheumatic disease patients on a yearly basis. Not only are patients with rheumatic diseases at higher risk of contracting influenza compared with the general population,[3] but also they suffer from greater morbidity and exhibit prolonged viral shedding,[4] and influenza vaccination is associated with reduced risk of morbidity and mortality in this population.[5] Patients ages 65 or older should receive a high-dose formulation, which aligns with the ACIP recommendations, where clinical studies have shown variable clinical and cost effectiveness (approximately $20 for standard dose vaccines vs approximately $50 dollars for high dose, without insurance, per Centers for Diseases Control and Prevention [CDC] 2020).[6] A randomized controlled trial assessed antibody responses to a standard-dose quadrivalent influenza vaccine compared with a high-dose trivalent inactivated formulation (HD-TIV) in patients with RA of mean age 61 years and found that those who received HD-TIV achieved superior immunogenicity.[7] High-dose influenza vaccine also has been shown to improve immunogenicity in solid organ transplant patients compared with standard dose.[8] Although there currently is no formal recommendation to administer high-dose influenza vaccines to rheumatic disease patients less than 50 years of age, these findings should be taken into consideration and prompt further studies, because they may be practice-changing.

Pneumococcal

Streptococcus pneumoniae is the leading cause of community-acquired pneumonia, and invasive disease is associated with a high mortality rate in the general population; this rate is even higher in patients with rheumatic diseases.[9] In the United States, pneumococcal vaccines are available as a 13-valent pneumococcal conjugate vaccine (PCV13) and a 23-valent pneumococcal polysaccharide vaccine (PPSV23). ACIP recommends the prime-boost vaccine strategy for pneumococcal vaccine series in immunocompromised patients, which includes a dose of PCV13 followed at least 8 weeks later by PPSV23, because this sequence has been shown to enhance antibody response compared with a single dose of PCV13 in patients with rheumatic diseases.[10] This strategy is included in the recommendations by the ACR, EULAR, and the European Society of Clinical Microbiology and Infectious Diseases. There are some nuances to this strategy, including specific recommendations for patients who have received PPSV23 prior to PCV13 (**Table 1**), often leading to patients with rheumatic diseases receiving the series incompletely. Despite these nuances, the prime-boost pneumococcal vaccine series should be given to all rheumatic disease patients contemplating starting or already on immunosuppressive medications.

Herpes Zoster

In immunocompetent persons, HZ is a common condition with incidence increasing significantly with age and is associated with substantial morbidity, including painful postherpetic neuralgia, among other complications. Vaccination against HZ is recommended for persons ages 50 and older. In patients with autoimmune and inflammatory diseases, the incidence of HZ is significantly higher, due to both underlying disease and immunosuppressive medications.[11] There are 2 available vaccines against HZ, the live zoster vaccine (LZV) and the recombinant zoster vaccine (RZV). RZV is a non-live recombinant subunit vaccine with a novel potent adjuvant, Food and Drug Administration (FDA)-approved in 2017, and now is the preferred HZ vaccine by ACIP. Rheumatology society recommendations are outdated, with the ACR recommending LZV be given prior to biologic therapy or tofacitinib for patients ages greater than or equal to 50 years, and EULAR encouraging rheumatologists to consider LZV administration in mildly immunosuppressed patients on a case-by-case basis, which often leaves providers unclear regarding best practices.

The clinical trials that led to RZV approval excluded patients with autoimmune diseases and patients receiving immunosuppressive medications; thus, administering RZV to rheumatic disease patients remains an area of uncertainty due to theoretic concern for disease flare and increased risk of injection site reactions and systemic symptoms as a result of the potent adjuvant used in the vaccine.[12,13] Given the increased incidence of HZ and its complications (including stroke[14]) and an increasing amount of evidence and clinical experience demonstrating acceptable safety of RZV in rheumatic disease patients,[15] RZV should be considered in rheumatic disease patients ages greater than or equal to 50 years, especially in patients receiving treatment with Janus kinase (JAK) inhibitors, where the risk is significantly higher compared with those treated with other biologic disease-modifying drugs.[16]

Herpes Papillomavirus

Human papillomavirus vaccine (HPV). is the most common sexually transmitted infection in the United States and is associated with cervical, vulvar, and vaginal cancer in women, penile cancer in men, and anal and oropharyngeal cancer in both men and women.[17] There is no treatment of HPV infection, further emphasizing the importance of this vaccine. ACIP recommends 3 vaccination with a 2-dose series for ages 9 through 14, and a 3-dose series if initiated between ages 15 years through 26 years;

Table 1
Important vaccines for patients with rheumatic diseases and considerations for administration

Vaccine	Indications for Rheumatic Disease Patients	Contraindications/ Considerations
Influenza		
Numerous inactivated formulations	• Yearly inactivated vaccine recommended for all patients • Patients ≥65 y should receive high-dose vaccine	Rituximab: ideally administer before start of therapy or as long after the first dose and 4 weeks prior to next dose, if possible. Methotrexate: consider holding 2 doses after vaccine administration, in inflammatory arthritis patients with quiescent disease
Live intranasal vaccine		Contraindicated in the setting of CDC recommended immunosuppressive thresholds (see **Box 1**)
Pneumococcal		
PPSV23	Prime-boost series recommended for all patients on immunosuppression: • Vaccine-naïve: PCV13 followed by PPSV23 ≥8 wk later • If <65 y at the start of series, repeat PPSV23 after 5 y. • All patients should receive a final dose of PPSV23 after age 65. • Previously vaccinated with PPSV23: PCV13 ≥ 1 y after PPSV23 • Patients need only 1 PCV13 in a lifetime.	Rituximab and methotrexate: administer before start of therapy, when possible.
PCV13		Efficacy may be reduced by abatacept and tofacitinib.
Herpes Zoster		
LZV	• ACR recommends LZV be given prior to biologic therapy or tofacitinib for RA patients ≥50 y. • EULAR recommends considering LZV administration in mildly immunosuppressed patients on a case-by-case basis.	Contraindicated in the setting of CDC-recommended immunosuppressive thresholds (see **Box 1**)

(continued on next page)

Table 1 (continued)		
Vaccine	Indications for Rheumatic Disease Patients	Contraindications/ Considerations
RZV	• No formal recommendations for administration	In light of an increasing amount of safety data, RZV should be recommended to patients with quiescent rheumatic disease, with informed decision making.
HPV		
9-valent formulation	• ACIP recommends 2-dose series for ages 9–14, and 3-dose series if initiated between 15–26; consider vaccinated ages 27–45 if not vaccinated previously. • 3-dose series recommended regardless of age in immunocompromised persons	Of particular importance in SLE patients

however, the 3-dose series is recommended regardless of age for immunocompromised persons.[18] HPV is of particular importance in patients with systemic lupus erythematosus (SLE), because this patient population experiences a higher incidence of HPV infection, are infected with more often high-risk subtypes, and are less likely to clear infection spontaneously, thus leading to higher rates of cervical and other cancers.[19] ACIP recommendations have been updated to include considering vaccinating adults ages 27 years through 45 years who have not been adequately vaccinated, while acknowledging that benefit in this population may be limited because the vaccine is most effective if received before HPV exposure; however, assessing HPV vaccine status in patients with rheumatic disease, especially patients with SLE, should be done regularly.

Other Vaccines

There are many other vaccines to consider in patients with rheumatic diseases; hepatitis B and tetanus vaccinations are highlighted. Hepatitis B virus is transmitted through blood and sexual contact, and chronic hepatitis B infection increases risk for cirrhosis and liver cancer. ACIP recommendations for adult hepatitis B vaccination are risk based rather than universal (but universally recommended for newborns within 24 hours of birth), and vaccination is recommended for adults with certain risk factors, including chronic liver disease (including hepatitis C, cirrhosis, alcoholic liver disease, and autoimmune hepatitis), HIV, diabetes, intravenous drug use, men having sex with men, dialysis, and health care work[20] Anyone seeking protection from hepatitis B also may be vaccinated. Assessing hepatitis B risk is an opportune time to ensure that screening for chronic hepatitis B (and hepatitis C) has been done, because this is recommended (hepatitis B surface antigen, core, and surface antibodies) by the American Association for the Study of Liver Diseases prior to initiation of any immunosuppressive medication.[21]

Tetanus, diphtheria, and pertussis (Tdap) vaccination is recommended for anyone who previously did not receive Tdap at or after age 11, followed by a booster of

Tdap or tetanus and diphtheria vaccine every 10 years.[6] There are no special recommendations for immunocompromised persons regarding routine Tdap vaccination.

EFFECT OF IMMUNOSUPPRESSION ON VACCINE EFFICACY

Treatment with both conventional and biologic DMARDs can pose challenges to vaccine administration because their use can have an impact on vaccine responses. Impact on vaccine efficacy is dependent on type of immunosuppressive agent or combination of agents as well as timing of vaccine administration in relation to dosing, which is pertinent for biologics. When possible, immunizations should be administered prior to planned immunosuppression, and there are some therapies for which this is more important (eg, rituximab). Although the effect of newer biologic classes (inhibitors of JAK, interleukin [IL]-6 and IL-17 targeted therapies, and so forth) on vaccine efficacy are still being learned about, there is a growing amount of data demonstrating a negative impact of rituximab as well as methotrexate on response to influenza and pneumococcal vaccines.

Conventional Synthetic Disease-Modifying Antirheumatic Drugs

Methotrexate

Although there are data to suggest that serologic response to seasonal inactivated influenza vaccine in patients with rheumatic diseases appears to offer sufficient protection from influenza and its complications,[5] it is known that methotrexate impairs influenza vaccine responses.[22] Park and colleagues[23] examined the impact on immunogenicity of holding methotrexate for 2 doses after administration of inactivated quadrivalent influenza vaccine. In a prospective, randomized parallel-group multicenter study of 320 patients with RA, 75.5% in the methotrexate-hold group achieved a satisfactory vaccine response compared with 54.5% in the group that continued methotrexate, with higher seroprotection rates against all 4 antigens. There was a trend toward more disease flares in the methotrexate-hold group; however, it was not statistically significant. These findings are likely to be practice-changing, and holding methotrexate for 2 doses after seasonal influenza vaccination is a recommendation I make to my patients who have stable/inactive chronic inflammatory arthritis.

Methotrexate decreases humoral response to both the pneumococcal conjugate and polysaccharide vaccines.[24,25] Both the ACR and EULAR guidelines counsel that vaccines should preferably be administered prior to initiation of immunosuppression; however, this not always is possible. At present, there are no formal recommendations to hold methotrexate for the pneumococcal vaccine series.

Other disease-modifying antirheumatic drugs

Aside from methotrexate, there is little evidence to suggest a negative impact of other DMARDs, such as hydroxychloroquine, sulfasalazine, or leflunomide, on vaccine responses.[26,27] It is unlikely that azathioprine reduces vaccine efficacy; however, there have been conflicting reports of response to influenza vaccine, with a study in renal transplant patients showing no negative impact from azathioprine,[28] whereas a study in patients with SLE demonstrated a trend toward decreased vaccine efficacy, as evidenced by fewer seroconversions and appropriate rises in hemagglutinin inhibition titers compared with SLE patients receiving hydroxychloroquine, prednisone, or no drug.[29] Mycophenolate reduces influenza vaccine responses, seroprotection rates, and seroconversion rates in renal transplant patients, and in SLE patients its use has been associated with reduced response to HPV vaccine compared with use of other DMARDs.[26] At present, there are no recommendations to hold DMARD therapy for administration of any nonlive vaccine.

Biologics

Rituximab

Of all the biologics, rituximab has been shown to have the most significant impact on vaccine responses across different rheumatic disease and has the most profound impact on influenza and pneumococcal vaccine responses. This effect is further reduced by concomitant use of methotrexate. In a study examining antibody response to pneumococcal vaccine in 88 RA patients receiving rituximab, abatacept or tocilizumab with or without methotrexate, only 10.3% of patients receiving rituximab and no patients receiving rituximab with methotrexate achieved a positive antibody response.[30] It is recommended by both ACR and EULAR to time vaccine administration accordingly. Specifically, for a patient planning to start or already receiving rituximab, influenza and pneumococcal vaccines should be given at least 6 months after administration and 4 weeks before the next course of B-cell–depleting therapy, when possible.[2,31] If timing influenza vaccine administration prior to rituximab dosing to maximize efficacy is not feasible, some protection against influenza is better than none at all, and influenza vaccine should be given regardless, taking into account potential for suboptimal response.

Inhibitors of tumor necrosis factor

Aside from B-cell–depleting biologics, such as rituximab, other biologic DMARDs have various impacts on vaccine responses. Tumor necrosis factor (TNF) inhibitors have little to no effect on antibody response to the pneumococcal vaccine series or influenza vaccines. A systematic review of 12 studies assessing the impact of immunosuppressive therapies on humoral response to pneumococcal and influenza vaccines in RA patients found no association between TNF inhibition and reduced vaccine responses,[32] and this has been demonstrated in numerous other studies.[25] Although this is reassuring, TNF inhibitors often are used with methotrexate, so impact of methotrexate on vaccine response in this setting must be considered.

Abatacept

There is little consistent evidence to date suggesting a negative impact of abatacept, a T-cell costimulation modulator approved for treatment of RA, juvenile idiopathic arthritis, and psoriatic arthritis, on vaccine responses; however, there have been case reports suggesting blunted response. As with other biologics, most studies have examined the drug's impact on influenza and pneumococcal vaccines. In the study discussed previously, by Crnkic Kapetanovi, and colleagues,[30] abatacept-treated RA patients receiving pneumococcal conjugate vaccine did exhibit impaired antibody responses compared with controls but to a lesser degree than the group receiving rituximab. In an analysis of 2 multicenter open-label substudies of abatacept in RA, patients receiving weekly subcutaneous abatacept mounted appropriate responses to both pneumococcal and influenza vaccines.[33]

Interleukin-6 inhibitors

There currently are 2 FDA-approved IL-6 inhibitors indicated for treatment of RA (tocilizumab and sarilumab) as well as for giant cell arteritis, juvenile idiopathic arthritis, and cytokine release syndrome from chimeric antigen receptor-T-cell therapy (tocilizumab). The most safety data exist for tocilizumab, because it was approved first (2010, in the United States) and to date there are no data to suggest any adverse impact of tocilizumab on vaccine responses; however, concomitant use of methotrexate may have an impact on vaccine responses.[34]

Janus kinase inhibitors

A growing number of JAK inhibitors are newer additions to the armamentarium of treatment options for rheumatic diseases, and most of the existing data on their impact on vaccine responses are with the agent tofacitinib. In a placebo-controlled study examining the effects of tofacitinib on pneumococcal and influenza vaccine immunogenicity in a group of 200 RA patients, Winthrop and colleagues[35] found that fewer tofacitinib-treated patients developed satisfactory responses to the pneumococcal polysaccharide vaccine (45.1% vs 68.4%, respectively) and pneumococcal titers also were lower with tofacitinib (and even lower if concomitant methotrexate). They observed similar rates of satisfactory influenza vaccine responses; however, fewer tofacitinib-treated patients developed protective influenza titers although overall effect was felt to be minimal.

Other biologics

There are numerous other newer targeted therapies, including inhibitors of IL-17 and IL-12/23, and there is a paucity of evidence to suggest these agents have a negative impact on vaccine responses. Small studies have shown no impact on immunogenic response to seasonal influenza vaccine and PPSV23 in the setting of anti–IL-17 therapy for treatment of inflammatory arthritis (secukinumab)[36] or in healthy persons (ixekizumab).[37]

Immunosuppression and live vaccines

In general, administration of live vaccines (yellow fever, varicella, measles, and mumps rubella) is contraindicated in the setting of immunosuppressive therapy, as defined by the CDC (**Box 1**), as well as biologic DMARDs. There are circumstances under which rheumatic disease patients need a live vaccine (job requirements, school requirements, and so forth), and experts recommend that any live vaccine be give 4 weeks prior to immunosuppressive treatment initiation. For patients already on biologic therapy, there are no formal recommendations of how long to hold therapy if live vaccine is needed and this has not been heavily studied. Experts recommend holding immunosuppression at least 1 month before and 1 month after vaccination.

Of interest are safety data regarding the measles, mumps, and rubella (MMR) vaccine and LZV, suggesting there may be exceptions to the rule. Evidence for potential safety of MMR administration is drawn from the pediatric rheumatic disease population, where several studies have demonstrated appropriate vaccine responses as well as safety of MMR vaccine in juvenile idiopathic arthritis patients receiving methotrexate, etanercept, and other biologics.[38,39]

Box 1
Centers for Disease Control and Prevention–defined immunosuppressive therapy during which live vaccine administration should be avoided

- Methotrexate $\geq$0.4 mg/kg/wk

- Azathioprine $\geq$3 mg/kg/d

- 6-mercaptopurine $\geq$1.5 mg/kg/d

- Glucocorticoid usage $\geq$2 weeks in doses equivalent to prednisone 20 mg/d or 2 mg/kg body weight

Adapted from Centers for Disease Control and Prevention (CDC). Vaccine Recommendations and Guidelines of the ACIP. Available at: https://www.cdc.gov/vaccines/hcp/acip-recs/general-recs/contraindications.html. Accessed Sept 2 2020.

Administration of the LZV in the setting of tofacitinib has been studied, through a post hoc analysis of a phase IIB/IV randomized study of methotrexate-inadequate responders receiving tofacitinib, 5 mg twice daily; tofacitinib, 5 mg twice daily plus methotrexate; or adalimumab plus methotrexate to treat RA.[40] Of the 1146 patients, 216 (18.8%) received LZV 28 days before initiation of study treatment. Although the study was not powered for comparisons between vaccinated and nonvaccinated groups, the data suggest that LZV is well tolerated in tofacitinib-treated RA patients. The Varicella Zoster Vaccine study, a blinded 1:1 randomized placebo-controlled trial of LZV in patients receiving TNF inhibitors, identified no new safety concerns.[41] With the introduction of the more effective RZV to prevent HZ, safety concerns surrounding LZV administration in rheumatic disease patients is less of an issue, however, still pertinent in regions with limited or no access to RZV.

EFFECT OF VACCINES ON RHEUMATIC DISEASE ACTIVITY

Ideally, immunizations should be administered during quiescent disease, and this is supported by ACR and EULAR recommendations. Despite studies showing no evidence for an association between influenza vaccination and disease flare in patients with chronic inflammatory arthritis or SLE,[42] patients' concerns for side effects or disease flare remain barriers to vaccine uptake. There are some circumstances where this consideration becomes more pertinent, and these are discussed.

As discussed previously, RZV was not heavily studied in patients with autoimmune or inflammatory diseases, and the vaccine's increased risk of local and systemic injection site reactions has left many practitioners and patients hesitant to give/receive RZV to patients with rheumatic diseases. Although more studies on efficacy and safety in this patient population are needed, results of several small studies have been encouraging. In the largest study to date, Stevens and colleagues[15] retrospectively analyzed 403 rheumatic disease patients who received RZV at a single center and observed a disease flare incidence of 6.7% after vaccination and that of side effects (soreness at the injection site, rash, fever, stomach ache, nausea, and flulike symptoms) was 12.7%, both less than the incidence reported in the clinical trials that led to RZV approval. Although larger, prospective studies are needed to confirm these observations, these data provide a framework for shared and informed decision making between health care provider and patient. At present, I strongly recommend RZV in my rheumatic disease patient population, as long as their underlying disease is quiescent, and after discussing the potential adverse effects.

Also of note is a reported increased risk of gout, observed in the pivotal RZV trials,[13] which also has been observed in the setting of other vaccines and felt to be related to activation of the NLRP3 inflammasome by the adjuvant systems employed in various vaccines.[43] Although this is of interest, gout flare risk appears to be low, and avoiding vaccine administration due to concern for gout flare is not recommended. Along these same lines, pneumococcal vaccination has been associated with systemic adverse reaction in patients with autoinflammatory diseases, in particular cryopyrin-associated periodic syndromes, and should be administered with caution in this patient population.[44]

SUMMARY

Patients with rheumatic diseases have an increased risk of infection, and there are many vaccines available in the armamentarium to lower the risk of vaccine-preventable infections and their complications. Every effort should be made to routinely assess vaccine status and ensure that recommended vaccines are up to date and administered prior to start of methotrexate and rituximab, when possible. Despite the known importance of routine vaccination in this vulnerable patient population, vaccine uptake remains low. Although there exist gaps in knowledge of vaccine efficacy in the setting of rheumatic diseases and immunosuppressive treatment, in particular, the newer biologics, and most of these recommendations are based on expert opinion/level C evidence, the information discussed in this article should provide a framework for rheumatologist and other health care providers to guide best practices and minimize infections in this at-risk population.

CLINICS CARE POINTS

- Seasonal flu vaccine should be actively recommended to all patients every year.
- The prime-boost pneumococcal vaccination method of administering PCV13 first followed by PPSV23 at least 8 weeks later should be given to all immunosuppressed rheumatic disease patients.
- Rituximab and methotrexate have the most significant impact on vaccine immunogenicity; influenza and pneumococcal vaccine administration should be timed prior to rituximab dosing and methotrexate held for 2 weeks after influenza vaccination when possible.
- The recombinant HZ vaccine has potential to cause injection site and systemic reactions, as well as rheumatic disease flare, but appears to be safe to administer and should be recommended, with informed decision making.

DISCLOSURE

C. Calabrese has consulted for AbBvie and consults and speaks for Sanofi-Regeneron.

REFERENCES

1. Singh JA, Saag KG, Bridges SL, et al. 2015 American College of Rheumatology Guideline for the treatment of rheumatoid arthritis. Arthritis Rheumatol 2016; 68(1):1–26.
2. Furer V, Rondaan C, Heijstek MW, et al. 2019 update of EULAR recommendations for vaccination in adult patients with autoimmune inflammatory rheumatic diseases. Ann Rheum Dis 2020;79(1):39–52.
3. Blumentals WA, Arreglado A, Napalkov P, et al. Rheumatoid arthritis and the incidence of influenza and influenza-related complications: a retrospective cohort study. BMC Musculoskelet Disord 2012;13(1):158.
4. Memoli MJ, Athota R, Reed S, et al. The Natural History of Influenza Infection in the Severely Immunocompromised vs Nonimmunocompromised Hosts. Clin Infect Dis 2014;58(2):214–24. https://doi.org/10.1093/cid/cit725.
5. Nakafero G, Grainge MJ, Myles PR, et al. Effectiveness of inactivated influenza vaccine in autoimmune rheumatic diseases treated with disease-modifying antirheumatic drugs. Rheumatology 2020;0:1–10. https://doi.org/10.1093/rheumatology/keaa078.
6. Freedman MS, Hunter P, Ault K, et al. Advisory committee on immunization practices recommended immunization schedule for adults aged 19 years or older — United States, 2020. MMWR Morb Mortal Wkly Rep 2020;69(5):133–5.
7. Colmegna I, Useche ML, Rodriguez K, et al. Immunogenicity and safety of high-dose versus standard-dose inactivated influenza vaccine in rheumatoid arthritis

patients: a randomised, double-blind, active-comparator trial. Lancet Rheumatol 2020;2(1):e14–23.

8. Natori Y, Shiotsuka M, Slomovic J, et al. A double-blind, randomized trial of high-dose vs standard-dose influenza vaccine in adult solid-organ transplant recipients. Clin Infect Dis 2018;66(11):1698–704.

9. Rákóczi É, Szekanecz Z. Pneumococcal vaccination in autoimmune rheumatic diseases. RMD Open 2017;3(2). https://doi.org/10.1136/rmdopen-2017-000484.

10. Nived P, Jönsson G, Settergren B, et al. Prime-boost vaccination strategy enhances immunogenicity compared to single pneumococcal conjugate vaccination in patients receiving conventional DMARDs, to some extent in abatacept but not in rituximab-treated patients. Arthritis Res Ther 2020;22(1):36.

11. Curtis JR, Xie F, Yang S, et al. Risk for herpes zoster in tofacitinib-treated rheumatoid arthritis patients with and without concomitant methotrexate and glucocorticoids. Arthritis Care Res 2019;71(9):1249–54.

12. Cunningham AL, Lal H, Kovac M, et al. Efficacy of the herpes zoster subunit vaccine in adults 70 years of age or older. N Engl J Med 2016;375(11):1019–32.

13. Lal H, Cunningham AL, Godeaux O, et al. Efficacy of an adjuvanted herpes zoster subunit vaccine in older adults. N Engl J Med 2015;372(22):2087–96.

14. Calabrese LH, Xie F, Yun H, et al. Herpes zoster and the risk of stroke in patients with autoimmune diseases. Arthritis Rheumatol 2017;69(2):439–46.

15. Stevens E, Weinblatt ME, Massarotti E, et al. Safety of the zoster vaccine recombinant adjuvanted in rheumatoid arthritis and other systemic rheumatic disease patients: a single center's experience with 400 patients. ACR Open Rheumatol 2020. https://doi.org/10.1002/acr2.11150. acr2.11150.

16. Winthrop KL. The emerging safety profile of JAK inhibitors in rheumatic disease. Nat Rev Rheumatol 2017;13(4):234–43.

17. Serrano B, Brotons M, Bosch FX, et al. Epidemiology and burden of HPV-related disease. Best Pract Res Clin Obstet Gynaecol 2018;47:14–26.

18. Meites E, Kempe A, Markowitz LE. Use of a 2-dose schedule for human papillomavirus vaccination — updated recommendations of the advisory committee on immunization practices. MMWR Morb Mortal Wkly Rep 2016;65(49):1405–8.

19. Mendoza-Pinto C, García-Carrasco M, Vallejo-Ruiz V, et al. Incidence of cervical human papillomavirus infection in systemic lupus erythematosus women. Lupus 2017;26(9):944–51.

20. Schillie S, Vellozzi C, Reingold A, et al. Prevention of hepatitis B virus infection in the United States: recommendations of the advisory committee on immunization practices. MMWR Recomm Rep 2018;67(1):1–31.

21. Terrault NA, Lok ASF, Mcmahon BJ, et al. Update on prevention, diagnosis, and treatment of chronic hepatitis B: AASLD 2018 Hepatitis B Guidance. Hepatology 2018;67(4):1560–99.

22. Ribeiro ACM, Guedes LKN, Moraes JCB, et al. Reduced seroprotection after pandemic H1N1 influenza adjuvant-free vaccination in patients with rheumatoid arthritis: implications for clinical practice. Ann Rheum Dis 2011;70(12):2144–7.

23. Park JK, Lee YJ, Shin K, et al. Impact of temporary methotrexate discontinuation for 2 weeks on immunogenicity of seasonal influenza vaccination in patients with rheumatoid arthritis: a randomised clinical trial. Ann Rheum Dis 2018;77(6):898–904.

24. Kapetanovic MC, Roseman C, Jönsson G, et al. Antibody response is reduced following vaccination with 7-valent conjugate pneumococcal vaccine in adult methotrexate-treated patients with established arthritis, but not those treated with tumor necrosis factor inhibitors. Arthritis Rheum 2011;63(12):3723–32.

25. Kapetanovic MC, Saxne T, Sjöholm AS, et al. Influence of methotrexate, TNF blockers and prednisolone on antibody responses to pneumococcal polysaccharide vaccine in patients with rheumatoid arthritis. Rheumatology 2006;45:106–11.

26. McMahan ZH, Bingham CO. Effects of biological and non-biological immunomodulatory therapies on the immunogenicity of vaccines in patients with rheumatic diseases. Arthritis Res Ther 2014;16(1):506.

27. Gabay C, Bel M, Combescure C, et al. Impact of synthetic and biologic disease-modifying antirheumatic drugs on antibody responses to the AS03-adjuvanted pandemic influenza vaccine: a prospective, open-label, parallel-cohort, single-center study. Arthritis Rheum 2011;63(6):1486–96.

28. Keshtkar-Jahromi M, Argani H, Rahnavardi M, et al. Antibody response to influenza immunization in kidney transplant recipients receiving either azathioprine or mycophenolate: A controlled trial. Am J Nephrol 2008;28(4):654–60.

29. Holvast B, Huckriede A, Wilschut J, et al. Safety and efficacy of influenza vaccination in systemic lupus erythematosus patients with quiescent disease. Ann Rheum Dis 2006;65(7):913–8.

30. Crnkic Kapetanovic M, Saxne T, Jönsson G, et al. Rituximab and abatacept but not tocilizumab impair antibody response to pneumococcal conjugate vaccine in patients with rheumatoid arthritis. Arthritis Res Ther 2013;15(5).

31. Rehnberg M, Brisslert M, Amu S, et al. Vaccination response to protein and carbohydrate antigens in patients with rheumatoid arthritis after rituximab treatment. Arthritis Res Ther 2010;12(3):R111.

32. Hua C, Barnetche T, Combe B, et al. Effect of methotrexate, anti-tumor necrosis factor α, and rituximab on the immune response to influenza and pneumococcal vaccines in patients with rheumatoid arthritis: a systematic review and meta-analysis. Arthritis Care Res 2014;66(7):1016–26.

33. Alten R, Bingham CO, Cohen SB, et al. Antibody response to pneumococcal and influenza vaccination in patients with rheumatoid arthritis receiving abatacept. BMC Musculoskelet Disord 2016;17(1):231.

34. Mori S, Ueki Y, Akeda Y, et al. Pneumococcal polysaccharide vaccination in rheumatoid arthritis patients receiving tocilizumab therapy. Ann Rheum Dis 2013; 72(8):1362–6.

35. Winthrop KL, Silverfield J, Racewicz A, et al. The effect of tofacitinib on pneumococcal and influenza vaccine responses in rheumatoid arthritis. Ann Rheum Dis 2016;75:687–95. https://doi.org/10.1136/annrheumdis-2014-207191.

36. Richi P, Martín MD, De Ory F, et al. Secukinumab does not impair the immunogenic response to the influenza vaccine in patients. RMD Open 2019;5(2):1018.

37. Gomez EV, Bishop JL, Jackson K, et al. Response to Tetanus and Pneumococcal Vaccination Following Administration of Ixekizumab in Healthy Participants. BioDrugs 2017;31(6):545–54.

38. Borte S, Liebert UG, Borte M, et al. Efficacy of measles, mumps and rubella revaccination in children with juvenile idiopathic arthritis treated with methotrexate and etanercept. Rheumatology 2009;48(2):144–8. https://doi.org/10.1093/rheumatology/ken436.

39. Heijstek MW, Kamphuis S, Armbrust W, et al. Effects of the live attenuated measles-mumps-rubella booster vaccination on disease activity in patients with juvenile idiopathic arthritis: A randomized trial. JAMA - J Am Med Assoc 2013; 309(23):2449–56.

40. Calabrese LH, Abud-Mendoza C, Lindsey SM, et al. Live zoster vaccine in patients with rheumatoid arthritis treated with tofacitinib with or without

methotrexate, or adalimumab with methotrexate: a post hoc analysis of data from a phase iiib/iv randomized study. Arthritis Care Res 2020;72(3):353–9.

41. Curtis J, Bridges S, Cofield S, et al. Results from a randomized controlled trial of the safety of the live varicella vaccine in TNF-treated patients - ACR meeting abstracts. Arthritis Rheumatol 2019;71(suppl 10). Available at: https://acrabstracts. org/abstract/results-from-a-randomized-controlled-trial-of-the-safety-of-the-live-varicella-vaccine-in-tnf-treated-patients/. [Accessed 28 June 2020].

42. Nakafero G, Grainge MJ, Myles PR, et al. Association between inactivated influenza vaccine and primary care consultations for autoimmune rheumatic disease flares: a self-controlled case series study using data from the Clinical Practice Research Datalink. Ann Rheum Dis 2019;78(8):1122–6.

43. Yokose C, Mccormick N, Chen C, et al. Risk of gout flares after vaccination: a prospective case cross-over study. Ann Rheum Dis 2019;78(11):1601–4.

44. Walker UA, Hoffman HM, Williams R, et al. Brief report: severe inflammation following vaccination against streptococcus pneumoniae in patients with cryopyrin-associated periodic syndromes. Arthritis Rheumatol 2016;68(2): 516–20.

Rheumatic Complications of Immune Checkpoint Inhibitors

Nilasha Ghosh, MD, Anne R. Bass, MD*

KEYWORDS

- Immune-related adverse events • Immune checkpoint inhibitors • Cancer
- Rheumatoid arthritis • Polymyalgia rheumatica • Myositis
- Disease-modifying antirheumatic drugs

KEY POINTS

- Immune checkpoint inhibitors can lead to autoimmune side effects called immune-related adverse events, which can mimic rheumatic diseases, such as rheumatoid arthritis, polymyalgia rheumatic, and polymyositis.
- Immune-related adverse events are common and can range in severity from asymptomatic to lethal.
- Due to the potential for high morbidity and mortality, prompt recognition of these events is important.

INTRODUCTION

Immune checkpoint inhibitors (ICIs) have dramatically changed how cancer has been treated in the past decade. These agents have been shown to provide significant survival benefits, especially after more traditional chemotherapies have failed. Immune checkpoint blockade allows T cells to overcome physiologic inhibitory mechanisms and mount an antitumor response[1–3] (**Fig. 1**). Although there are several checkpoint inhibitors under study and in production, there are 3 main classes of ICIs at this time, those targeting cytotoxic T-lymphocyte–associated protein-4 (CTLA-4), programmed cell death protein 1 (PD-1) or its ligand, and programmed death ligand 1 (PD-L1).

ICIs have been approved for the treatment of many malignancies, including melanoma, non–small cell lung cancer, renal cell carcinoma, and urothelial tumors (**Table 1**). They also have been approved for the treatment of tumors with mismatch repair (MMR) defects and/or a high mutational burden, regardless of the organ involved.[4,5] These tumors produce high levels of neoantigens, resulting in increased

This article originally appeared in the Medical Clinics of North America, Volume 105, Issue 2, March 2021.
Hospital for Special Surgery, Weill Cornell Medicine, New York, NY, USA
* Corresponding author. 535 East 70th Street, New York, NY 10021.
E-mail address: bassA@hss.edu

Rheum Dis Clin N Am 48 (2022) 411–428
https://doi.org/10.1016/j.rdc.2022.02.002
rheumatic.theclinics.com

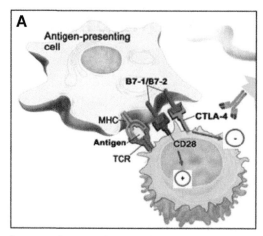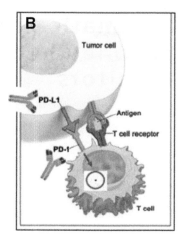

Fig. 1. Mechanism of action of ICIs.(*A*) Within the lymph node, an antigen is presented to a naive T cell receptor (TCR). CD28 on the T-cell binding to B7 provides the second signal needed to fully activate the T cell. CTLA-4 is a negative regulator that competes with CD28 to bind to B7 to turn the T cell off preventing overactivation. Antibodies to CTLA-4 block this inhibitory step, allowing for continued T-cell activation. (*B*) A cytotoxic T cell binds to a cancer cell's surface antigen via the TCR without the need for a second signal. PD-1 binding to PD-L1 on the target cell sends an inhibitory signal to the T cell to turn the cell off. Antibodies that block either PD-1 or PD-L1 block this inhibition. (For the National Cancer Institute Q 2019. *Adapted from*: Terese Winslow LLC, with permission. U.S. Govt, has certain rights.)

immunogenicity and sensitivity to ICIs. ICIs can be used alone, in combination, and/or in conjunction with conventional chemotherapy, radiotherapy, or surgery. Although they generally are used in patients with metastatic (stage IV) cancer, they increasingly are used as adjuvant therapy in patients with locally advanced cancers (stage III).

Although ICIs can effectively treat some cancers, ICI-induced T-cell activation can lead to autoimmune side effects, termed *immune-related adverse events* (*irAEs*).[6] The mechanisms underlying irAEs are not well understood, but activated cytotoxic T cells seem to play a direct role in some irAEs, such as myositis, whereas other irAEs appear to be antibody mediated, such as bullous pemphigoid.[6]

IrAEs occur in 80% to 90% of patients and can affect multiple organ systems in the body, including the skin, gastrointestinal (GI) tract, lungs, endocrine organs, and heart (**Table 2**). Approximately 5% of patients develop rheumatic complications, such as inflammatory arthritis.[6,7] Tumor type does not significantly influence which organs are targeted by irAE, but the specific ICI treatment does. For example, thyroid dysfunction and arthralgias are more common with PD-1 and PD-L1 blockade, whereas colitis and hypophysitis are more common with CTLA-4 blockade. The frequency and severity of irAEs are highest with combination therapy (anti–CTLA-4 plus anti–PD-1).[8] Within organ systems, irAE manifestations can vary from patient to patient. For example, skin involvement can manifest as vitiligo, lichenoid reactions, psoriasis, bullous pemphigoid, or Stevens-Johnson syndrome. Endocrine manifestations also are varied, including thyroiditis, leading to both hyperthyroidism and hypothyroidism, hypophysitis, type 1 diabetes mellitus, or adrenal insufficiency. IrAE severity is graded using the Common Terminology Criteria for Adverse Events (CTCAE) system and ranges from mild (grade 1), to moderate (grade 2), to severe and generally requiring hospitalization (grade 3), to life-threatening (grade 4), and to death (grade 5).[9] In the GI tract, for example, patients can have an increased number of daily bowel movements (grade 1) or frank colitis with perforation (grade 4 or 5). At present, biomarkers are lacking

Table 1
Food and Drug Administration–approved indications for immune checkpoint inhibitors

	Brand Name	Target	Food and Drug Administration Approval Year	Cancers Approved for Drug Use
Ipilimumab	Yervoy	CTLA-4	2011	Melanoma, renal cell carcinoma, colorectal cancer
Nivolumab	Opdivo	PD-1	2014	Melanoma, non–small cell lung cancer, small cell lung cancer, renal cell carcinoma, Hodgkin lymphoma, head and neck squamous cell cancer, urothelial carcinoma, colorectal cancer, hepatocellular carcinoma, esophageal cancer
Pembrolizumab	Keytruda	PD-1	2014	Melanoma, non–small cell lung cancer, small cell lung cancer, renal cell carcinoma, Hodgkin lymphoma, large B-cell lymphoma, gastric cancer, esophageal cancer, cervical cancer, Merkel cell carcinoma, head and neck squamous cell cancer, urothelial carcinoma, bladder cancer, colorectal cancer, hepatocellular carcinoma, advanced MSI-H/dMMR
Cemiplimab	Libtayo	PD-1	2018	Cutaneous squamous cell carcinoma
Avelumab	Bavencio	PD-L1	2017	Merkel cell carcinoma, urothelial carcinoma, renal cell carcinoma
Atezolizumab	Tecentriq	PD-L1	2016	Urothelial carcinoma, non–small -cell lung cancer, small cell lung cancer, bladder cancer, breast cancer, hepatocellular carcinoma
Durvalumab	Imfinzi	PL-LI	2017	Urothelial carcinoma, non–small lung cancer, small cell lung cancer

Abbreviations: MSI-H, microsatellite instability–high; dMMR, deficient MMR.

to predict the type and severity of irAE that an individual patient experiences, so close monitoring is of the essence. A majority of irAEs typically occur in the first 3 months after ICI initiation; however, irAEs can occur much earlier, within days of ICI initiation, to months after ICI discontinuation.[10,11] Fatal irAEs tend to occur soon after ICI initiation but they also can have a delayed or insidious onset.[12]

Although irAEs sometimes can result in significant morbidity or even mortality, they are associated with better cancer responses to ICI.[13] Early studies showed that melanoma patients who developed vitiligo after anti–CTLA-4 or anti–PD-1 had a significant survival benefit.[14,15] Later studies have shown a similar benefit from irAEs in general, especially in patients treated with anti–PD-1 or anti–PD-L1 agents.[13,16]

Because controlled trials to guide irAE management still are lacking, guidelines borrow from the literature on de novo autoimmune diseases, such as rheumatoid arthritis or inflammatory bowel disease, and rely heavily on corticosteroids and tumor necrosis factor inhibitors (TNFis), in refractory cases. Abatacept (CTLA-4 Ig), a CTLA-4 agonist used for the treatment of rheumatoid arthritis, generally is avoided because its mode of action is directly contrary to that of the ICI ipilimumab (anti–CTLA-4), raising concerns that it would abrogate the antitumor effects of ICI. It has been used, however, in a case of refractory and life-threatening ICI myocarditis.[17]

In this article, the authors review rheumatic irAEs that may be encountered in general medicine practice. A guiding principle is that early recognition and treatment of irAEs are important in order to minimize morbidity and mortality.

Table 2
Medications used in the management of immune-related adverse events

Drug (Target)	Onset of Action	Toxicity	Monitoring
NSAIDS	<1 d	GI Renal HTN Hepatitis	Baseline creatinine, Periodic creatinine for chronic use
Corticosteroids	<1 d	Infection Weight gain Osteoporosis Diabetes Hypertension Osteonecrosis Emotional lability	Baseline bone density, q2–3 y for chronic use BMP glucose or HgA1c for chronic use
Hydroxychloroquine	2–3 mo	Retinal pigmentation Neuropathy Myopathy, cardiomyopathy Skin pigmentation	Yearly eye examination
Sulfasalazine	2–3 mo	Sulfa allergy Headache GI Hematological Proteinuria Liver test abnormality	CBC, LFT, U/A 1 mo after initiation, then every 3–4 mo
Methotrexate	2–3 mo	Infection Mucosal ulcers Cytopenias Liver test abnormality, cirrhosis Pulmonary fibrosis	CBC, LFTs monthly × 3, then every 3–4 mo
Mycophenolate mofetil	1–3 mo	Infection GI Cytopenias	CBC, LFTs monthly × 3, then every 3–4 mo
TNFis[a]	<1 mo	Infection Multiple sclerosis Neuropathy Drug-induced lupus Psoriasis Rash	Baseline CBC, CMP, hepatitis B sAg, hepatitis B cAb, Quantiferon TBG CBC, LFTs 3 mo after initiation
IL-6R inhibitors [b]	<1 mo	Infection Cytopenias Liver test abnormalities Hyperlipidemia Intestinal perforation	CBC, LFTs monthly × 3, then every 3–4 mo Baseline lipids, retest 8 wk later
IVIG	<1 mo	Fluid overload Aseptic meningitis	IgA (evaluate for deficiency)
Rituximab (anti-CD20 B cell)	2–3 mo	Infection Infusion reactions Neutropenia Hypogammaglobulinemia PML	CBC 2–4 mo after infusion, CBC and quantitative immunoglobulins before each cycle

Abbreviations: BMP, basic metabolic panel; cAb, core antibody; CBC, complete blood count; HgA1c, Hemoglobin A1c; IgA, Immunoglobulin A; IVIG, Intravenous immunoglobulin; LFT, liver function test; QuantiFERON TB-Gold, TB Interferon-Gamma Release Assay; sAg, surface antigen; U/A, urinanalysis.
   [a] Infliximab, adalimumab, certolizumab, golimumab, etanercept.
   [b] Tocilizumab, sarilumab.

IMMUNE CHECKPOINT INHIBITORS IN PATIENTS WITH PREEXISTING AUTOIMMUNE DISEASE

There have been several retrospective studies evaluating the outcomes of ICI in patients with preexisting autoimmune disease. In general, approximately 75% of autoimmune disease patients have an irAE after ICI treatment, half an exacerbation of their autoimmune disease, one-third a de novo irAE, and some both. IrAE rates are lower in patients on immunosuppression at the time of ICI initiation, but cancer responses to the ICI also are lower in those patients.[18] Therefore, the authors recommend discontinuing or lowering the dose of immunosuppression prior to ICI initiation if the autoimmune disease itself is not life-threatening.

APPROACH TO THE PATIENT WITH MUSCULOSKELETAL COMPLAINTS AFTER IMMUNE CHECKPOINT INHIBITORS

When patients present with musculoskeletal pain after ICI treatment, the first step is to determine which organ is affected: joint, tendon, enthesis (the site where tendons or ligaments insert on bone), muscle, or nerve. If the joints are affected, then the number of joints and their distribution and symmetry can help characterize the arthritis phenotype as rheumatoid arthritis-like, spondyloarthropathy-like, polymyalgia rheumatica (PMR)–like, or a monoarthritis that could represent activated osteoarthritis (**Fig. 2**). Some patients have joint pain without joint swelling, characterized as arthralgia.

It also is important to document the severity of irAE symptoms because this guides the choice of therapy and whether the ICI should be held or discontinued. In addition to assigning an irAE grade (arthritis generally is graded 1–3), some kind of numerical disease activity score is helpful to monitor patients' response to therapy. The simplest is to document the patients' global assessment of arthritis activity on a visual analog scale (VAS) from 0 to 10 as well as the provider's VAS 0 to 10. The duration of morning stiffness (in minutes or hours) also is a useful marker of disease activity. In patients with frank arthritis, the number of tender and swollen joints also should be documented. The clinical disease activity index (CDAI)[19] is the sum of the tender and swollen joints (28-joint count) and patient and physician arthritis activity scores on a VAS: 0 to 10 is mild disease activity, 11 to 22 moderate, and greater than 22 high disease activity. The CDA provides a more nuanced assessment of arthritis disease activity than irAE grade and can be useful to track response to therapy from visit to visit.[19]

A targeted rheumatology review of systems can help screen for new conditions associated with musculoskeletal pain. The presence of psoriasis may point to a spondyloarthropathy, whereas dryness of the eyes or mouth, oral or nasal ulcers,

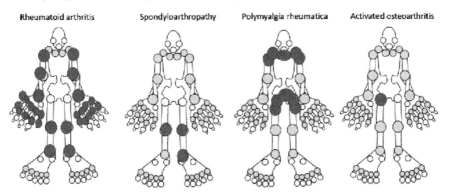

Fig. 2. Examples of ICI-associated musculoskeletal phenotypes (blue dots indicate tender and/or swollen joints). (Figure reproduced and modified with permission from CaRE Arthritis.)

photosensitivity, or Raynaud phenomenon might suggest a connective tissue disease, like sicca syndrome (similar to Sjögren disease) or lupus. Lupus-like conditions, however, are uncommon in the context of ICI treatment. A personal or family history of autoimmunity, such as rheumatoid arthritis, psoriasis, psoriatic arthritis, inflammatory bowel disease, or uveitis, may point to one of those conditions being induced or unmasked by ICI.

Radiographic imaging is important especially in patients presenting with only 1 or 2 painful joints, in order to rule out underlying osteoarthritis or metastatic disease. Avascular necrosis also should be considered, especially in patients who have received high doses of corticosteroids for treatment of nonmusculoskeletal irAEs. Because back pain is uncommon in ICI arthritis, patients presenting with new and significant primarily axial complaints always should undergo imaging, often with magnetic resonance imaging (MRI), to rule out metastasis and/or pathologic fracture. The authors recommend hand radiographs to rule out erosions, particularly in patients with an rheumatoid arthrisit–like presentation, and of the knees if they are disproportionately affected. Normal radiographs, however, do not rule out the presence of an inflammatory arthropathy. Ultrasound of the joints can be used to identify synovitis when the physical examination is hard to interpret or to localize effusions for the purpose of joint aspiration.

Joint aspiration provides an opportunity to assess the degree of joint inflammation, rule out ICI-unrelated crystal disease, rule out infection (particularly if only 1 joint is affected), and inject with corticosteroids, if clinically indicated. The authors recommend referral to a rheumatologist if the patient has significant arthritis, for early consideration of steroid-sparing agents. Similarly, patients who are unable to taper corticosteroids within a month of treatment, even to a low dose (<10-mg prednisone equivalent), benefit from rheumatology consultation in order to consider additional therapies.

TREATMENT OVERVIEW

In general, the treatment of rheumatic irAEs is tailored to the organ system affected and the severity/grade of the irAE. Specific irAE treatment is outlined later, but some general principals follow. Grade 1 irAEs generally can be managed with symptom-directed therapies, such as analgesics or nonsteroidal anti-inflammatory drugs (NSAIDS), local injections if indicated, and, if necessary, low-dose prednisone, generally 10 mg or less. ICIs can be continued in patients with grade 1 irAE. For grade 2 irAE, higher doses of corticosteroids generally are required, and ICIs may be temporarily held. There is a low threshold for initiating steroid-sparing agents for rheumatic irAEs because they often persist, and patients can experience side effects related to long-term use of corticosteroids. Some of the disease-modifying antirheumatic drugs (DMARDs) that are used to manage irAEs are listed in **Table 3**. Mild but slow-acting steroid-sparing DMARDs include hydroxychloroquine and sulfasalazine, whereas more potent slow-acting agents include methotrexate and mycophenolate mofetil. In patients with grade 3 irAEs or patients with grade 2 irAEs who are unable to taper corticosteroids, biologic DMARDs are an attractive choice because of their relatively rapid onset of action. TNFis, in particular infliximab, now are standard of care for the management of steroid refractory ICI-induced colitis, and their early introduction in that setting is associated with a faster resolution of symptoms and a reduced risk of infection compared with high-dose corticosteroids alone.[20–22] The use of TNFis for the management of ICI arthritis has been described in several cohorts,[23,24] but large published series documenting their overall effectiveness and safety in comparison to other approaches are lacking.

The use of immunosuppressive agents to control irAEs might be presumed to counteract the beneficial effects of ICI treatment on cancers but this has been difficult to demonstrate, perhaps because irAEs themselves are associated with improved

Table 3
Approach to the management of rheumatological immune-related adverse events

	Clinical Examination	Testing	Treatment			
			Grade 1	Grade 2	Grade 3–4	
Arthritis	Look for swelling of small joints (MCP, PIP, wrists), tendons (eg, at the wrists, patella, quadriceps, triceps)	CBC ESR CRP RF CCP ANA	NSAIDS, Intraarticular injection Prednisone 5–10 mg if needed If unable to taper steroids, consider hydroxychloroquine, sulfasalazine	NSAIDS, Intraarticular injection Prednisone 10–30 mg If unable to taper steroids, consider hydroxychloroquine, sulfasalazine, methotrexate, TNFi, IL-6Ri	NSAIDS, Intraarticular injection Prednisone 30–60 mg If unable to taper steroids quickly, consider TNFi, IL-6Ri. MTX	
	Extra-articular features (eg, psoriasis)		Continue ICI	Hold ICI, rechallenge when prednisone 10 mg or less	Hold ICI	
PMR	Pain on ROM shoulders and hips Evaluate for signs of GCA (headache, temporal artery tenderness)	CBC ESR CRP RF CCP	NSAIDS, Subacromial bursa injection Prednisone 5–20 mg daily If unable to taper steroids, consider hydroxychloroquine, MTX	NSAIDS Prednisone 20–40 mg If unable to taper steroids, consider MTX, IL-6Ri	NSAIDS, Prednisone 40–60 mg If unable to taper steroids, consider IL-6Ri	
			Continue ICI	Hold ICI	Hold ICI	
Activated OA	Pain in joint previously affected by OA, usually hip or knee	X-ray Joint aspiration to rule out inflammatory arthritis, crystal disease	NSAIDS, Intraarticular steroid injection (US guided in the case of the hip)	NSAIDS, Intraarticular injection (US guided in the case of the hip) Consider prednisone 5–10 mg daily Consider orthopedic referral	NSAIDS, Intraarticular injection (US guided in the case of the hip) Consider prednisone 10–20 mg daily Consider orthopedic referral	

(continued on next page)

Table 3
(continued)

	Clinical Examination	Testing	Treatment		
			Grade 1	Grade 2	Grade 3–4
Sicca	Dry oral mucosa, parotid gland swelling, gritty sensation in eyes (The presence of blistering or ulceration suggests pemphigoid not sicca.)	CBC, ESR, CRP, ANA, RF, SSA (Ro), SSB (La) antibodies	Biotin rinse Cevimeline or pilocarpine Continue ICI	Prednisone 10–30 mg daily Hold ICI; may be able to resume once steroid dose is tapered low enough	Prednisone 1 mg/kg Hold ICI
Myositis	Muscle, joint and neurologic examination, assess for dysphagia and dysphonia, extraocular muscle function Skin examination (consider dermatomyositis)	CK, troponin, transaminases, CBC, ESR, CRP, antistriated muscle, acetylcholine receptor, and myositis antibody panel Echocardiogram and EKG to screen for concomitant myocarditis. NIFs if evidence of respiratory compromise, swallowing evaluation if dysphagia Consider EMG, MRI, and/or muscle biopsy	If myalgia only, NSAIDs, can be used If CK elevation but no muscle weakness, prednisone 10–20 mg daily If muscle weakness, then treat as grade 2 Continue ICI	Prednisone 0.5–1 mg/kg daily Rheumatology and/or neurology consultation Cardiology consult if troponin elevation Hold ICI, may consider re-challenge if no cardiac or bulbar involvement	Methylprednisolone 1 g IV and then 1 mg/kg, consider IVIG or PLEX Consider methotrexate, azathioprine, mycophenolate mofetil If refractory, consider rituximab. Rheumatology and/or neurology consultation Cardiology consult if troponin elevated Discontinue ICI

	Symptoms	Workup	Mild	Moderate	Severe
Eosinophilic fasciitis	Skin thickening and tethering Pain in limbs Loss of range of motion of the joints due to tightening of the fascia Sparing of the hands and face	CBC with eosinophil count, ESR, CRP, CPK Consider MRI Consider deep skin biopsy	Consider 0.5 mg– 1 mg/kg prednisone daily with taper Consider phototherapy Continue ICI	Consider 1 mg/kg prednisone Consider addition of DMARD, such as methotrexate, mycophenolate mofetil, dapsone Hold ICI	Pulse-dose steroids DMARD therapy, consider cyclophosphamide Rheumatology and dermatology consultation Hold ICI
GCA	New headache, loss of vision, jaw claudication, temporal tenderness, scalp tenderness, neck pain, symptoms of PMR	CBC with diff, CMP, ESR, CRP c-ANCA Temporal artery biopsy Bone densitometry	Not applicable/NA	1mg/kg prednisone daily with taper Calcium–vitamin D Consider bisphosphonate if on steroid monotherapy Strongly consider IL-6Ri Hold ICI	ER/hospital admission Pulse-dose steroids Strongly consider IL-6Ri, Calcium/vitamin D Consider bisphosphonate if on steroid monotherapy Rheumatology, ophthalmology consult Hold ICI
Sarcoidosis	Fatigue, weight loss, malaise, cough, myalgias, weakness, arthralgias or arthritis, rash	CBC with diff CMP, including calcium ESR CRP CPK, ACE level Chest radiograph Consider skin or transbronchial biopsy	No treatment necessary unless symptomatic NSAIDs Topical steroids Hydroxychloroquine Consider prednisone 5–10 mg for joint pain or other mild symptoms Continue ICI	Consider prednisone 10–30 mg daily Topical steroids Hold ICI; may be resume ICI once steroid dose is low enough	Consider 0.5–1 mg/kg prednisone or higher Consultation with rheumatology, dermatology or pulmonology Hold ICI

Abbreviations: ACE, angiotensin-converting enzyme; ANA, anti-nuclear antigen; CK or CPK, creatine phosphokinase; CMP, complete metabolic panel; CRP, C-reactive protein; diff, differential; EKG, electrocardiogram; ER, emergency room; ESR, erythrocyte sedimentation ratio; IV, intravenous; MCP, metacarpophalangeal; MRI, magnetic resonance imaging; N/A, not applicable; NIF, negative inspiratory force; OA, osteoarthritis; PIP, proximal interphalangeal; PLEX, plasmapharesis; ROM, range of motion; US, ultrasound.

survival.[13,15,16] One retrospective study of patients treated for ICI-induced hypophysitis demonstrated a marked reduction in survival in those treated with high-dose compared with low-dose corticosteroids.[25] In cases of TNFi, retrospective studies have produced conflicting results in regard to their impact on survival.[22,26] Although patients with ICI-induced colitis often require only a single dose of infliximab, patients with ICI arthritis tend to have persistent symptoms over months,[27] so the long-term safety of these agents is important, particularly in this setting. Preclinical studies suggest that the short-term use of TNFi may, if anything, be beneficial in combating tumors.[28]

Rheumatic Immune-related Adverse Events

Inflammatory arthritis

Joint pains (arthralgia) occur commonly in ICI-treated patients. A meta-analysis of clinical trials estimated the incidence (95% CI) of arthralgia to be 5% (3%–9%) with anti–CTLA-4, 8% (7%–11%) with anti–PD-(L)1, and 11% with the combination.[8] A 3-way head to head ICI trial also showed that joint pain is most frequent in patients getting combination therapy and least frequent with anti–CTLA-4.[1] Inflammatory arthritis (joint pain accompanied by joint swelling) is less common than arthralgia; however, estimates are hard to come by because joint swelling rarely has been documented in the context of these clinical trials. In 1 large prospective ICI cancer cohort, 3.8% of patients were referred to a rheumatologist for inflammatory arthritis.[29] This also may be an underestimate, however, because arthritis symptoms sometimes are ignored, especially if a patient is experiencing a potentially life-threatening irAE, such as colitis. In addition, treatment of nonarticular irAEs with corticosteroids or TNFis can treat the arthritis as well, and the arthritis then may go undetected.

ICI arthritis typically occurs in the first several months after ICI initiation but can occur more than a year after ICI initiation. In 1 cohort of 30 ICI arthritis patients, median (interquartile range) time of onset was 3 (1.3–12) months after ICI initiation.[23] There can be a very long delay between ICI arthritis onset and referral to a rheumatologist, as shown by Cappelli and colleagues.[23] In that cohort, patients with knee arthritis generally were referred within 1 month to 2 months whereas there was a median delay of a year before referral of patients with arthritis of the small joints of the hands. Oncologists have become more aware of ICI arthritis in recent years, however.

Just as inflammatory arthritis can take different forms in the non-ICI setting (eg, rheumatoid arthritis, psoriatic arthritis, or ankylosing spondylitis), ICI arthritis also has a variety of presentations (see **Fig. 1**). Approximately two-thirds of ICI arthritis patients have a rheumatoid arthritis–like presentation with symmetric involvement of the MCP and PIP joints and wrists as well as larger joints.[6,23,30,31] Some patients have joint pain (arthralgia) and morning stiffness but no objective joint swelling. Another phenotype is a large joint arthritis, affecting the knees in particular, sometimes with accompanying tenosynovitis (swelling in the tendon sheath) or enthesitis (pain where tendons insert on bone) and, rarely, with concomitant psoriasis. Tenosynovitis/enthesitis also can occur in the absent of arthritis. Large joint arthritis seems more common after combination ICI than ICI monotherapy.[23] Although the large joint phenotype is reminiscent of spondyloarthropathies, patients generally are HLA-B27 negative.[32]

Laboratory testing in patients with ICI arthritis sometimes, but not always, shows elevated inflammatory markers. Joint fluid is inflammatory but there are no unique synovial fluid findings in this condition. The frequency of rheumatoid factor (RF) and anticyclic citrullinated peptide antibody (CCP) varies from cohort to cohort. In a series of ICI arthritis patients from Baltimore, only 3% were seropositive,[23] whereas seropositivity was approximately 30% in a Munich cohort.[32] In a systematic review of case series and case reports, 9% of patients with ICI arthritis were RF positive and/or CCP positive.[30] Whether these patients had preexisting autoantibodies or whether they seroconverted after ICI initiation is not known. ICIs have been shown to induce autoantibody seroconversion, including RF and CCP, but in 1 study of 121 patients treated with ipilimumab (anti–CTLA-4), none of the 3 patients who developed RF/CCP antibodies developed ICI arthritis, whereas the 3 patients developed arthralgia or arthritis remained seronegative.[33]

Thirty years ago, Gregersen and colleagues[34] demonstrated an association between rheumatoid arthritis and the shared epitope, a 5–amino acid motif found in certain HLA-DRB1 alleles. Later, the genetic association with rheumatoid arthritis was shown to be limited to CCP-positive patients, in particular smokers.[35] In a study of 26 patients of European descent with ICI arthritis from the Baltimore cohort, heterozygosity for the shared epitope was twice as common as in healthy controls (and comparable to patients with RA), even though only 4 of the patients were seropositive (2 CCP and 2 RF).[36] This suggests there are both shared and unshared mechanisms underlying ICI arthritis and RA, and this ultimately may add to understanding of rheumatoid arthritis pathogenesis. A gene signature that has been shown to be upregulated in cancer patients treated with nivolumab (anti–PD-1) also has been shown to be up-regulated in patients with active RA,[37] again suggesting some shared pathophysiologic mechanisms.

Approach to the patient History and physical examination should be performed to determine the particular joints that are affected and disease severity. The CTCAE grading system defines grade 1 arthritis as mild pain with inflammation, erythema, or joint swelling; grade 2 as moderate pain associated with signs of inflammation, erythema, or joint swelling, limiting instrumental activities of daily living (ADLs); and grade 3 as severe pain associated with signs of inflammation, erythema, or joint swelling, irreversible joint damage, limiting self-care ADLs (CTCAE).[9] As noted previously, measuring arthritis activity using the CDAI is helpful in measuring response to treatment.[19]

Laboratory testing can corroborate the clinical assessment of disease activity, including a complete blood cell count (CBC), C-reactive protein (CRP), and an erythrocyte sedimentation rate (ESR). Creatinine kinase (CK) testing is useful to rule out concomitant myositis. The authors generally test for CCP, RF, and antinuclear antibody (ANA). Testing for hepatitis B and hepatitis C and screening for tuberculosis exposure are useful at baseline, in case a patient ultimately requires DMARDs, such as methotrexate, or a TNFi. Radiographs or ultrasound of the hands should be performed in patients with small joint involvement to look for evidence of erosive disease. Many patients have prominent knee joint involvement and baseline radiographs of the knees also can be useful in that setting.

Treatment One of the distinguishing characteristics of ICI arthritis is its tendency to persist.[27] For this reason, DMARDs often are added early on in the course of treatment, even if symptoms are not severe, in order to spare patients long-term treatment with corticosteroids.

The overall approach to treatment is summarized. Grade 1 arthritis sometimes can be managed with NSAIDs and intraarticular steroid injections but may require the addition of low-dose oral corticosteroids (prednisone 5–10 mg daily or the equivalent). ICIs generally can be continued in this setting. If corticosteroids cannot be tapered after 1 month to 2 months, a mild DMARD, such as hydroxychloroquine or sulfasalazine, can be considered. These agents take 2 months to 3 months to have their effect but may be steroid sparing. In 1 series of 11 ICI arthritis patients treated with hydroxychloroquine and corticosteroids, 7 had control of their symptoms on treatment with this regimen.[38] Grade 2 arthritis may require higher doses of corticosteroids, up to 30 mg daily, and temporary holding if ICI. If corticosteroids cannot be tapered to 10 mg daily within 2 to 3 weeks, the authors generally add a steroid-sparing DMARD, which could include hydroxychloroquine, sulfasalazine, methotrexate, or a TNFi. Grade 3 arthritis requires treatment with high-dose corticosteroids. If symptoms are not controlled easily within 1 week to 2 weeks, the authors recommend treatment with a TNFi because of their rapid onset of action. Methotrexate can be added if there is only a partial response but takes 2 months to 3 months to have its effect. Patients who are refractory to TNFi can be switched to an interleukin (IL)-6R blocker, such as tocilizumab or sarilumab. In a published series of 3 ICI arthritis patients treated with tocilizumab, all had a clinical response to the drug, but 2 of 3 had cancer progression.[39] For this reason, the authors generally do not use IL-6R blockade as first-line therapy.

Polymyalgia Rheumatica

In the authors' systematic literature review of case series and case reports of ICI-associated musculoskeletal complaints, 78/372 (21%) had symptoms consistent with PMR.[30] As with PMR outside the ICI setting, ICI-associated PMR sometimes can be associated with some hand pain and swelling, suggesting some overlap with RA, and occasionally patients have a positive RF or CCP.[40] A diagnosis of ICI-associated PMR is a clinical one, based on the distribution of joint pain and stiffness (shoulders, neck, hips, thighs, and low back [see **Fig. 2**]). Acute-phase reactants may or may not be elevated.[40] As with patients with ICI-associated arthritis, the authors generally send a CBC, CK ESR, CRP, RF, and CCP. Given proximal limb involvement in ICI-associated PMR, it is important to consider myositis in the differential diagnosis. In contrast to patients with PMR, patients with myositis typically complain of weakness, which may be demonstrated on examination, and CK is elevated.

A majority of patients with ICI-associated PMR respond to corticosteroids alone but in 1 large case series, approximately half of the patients required more than 20 mg of prednisone daily,[40] more than typically is required for PMR. In the non-ICI setting, PMR can be associated with giant cell arteritis (GCA) in a small percentage of patients. GCA rarely has been described in patients treated with ICI,[41,42] even without elevated inflammatory markers, so it is important to ask any patient with symptoms of ICI-associated PMR whether they have cranial symptoms, such as temporal headache, scalp sensitivity, or jaw claudication. The presence of these symptoms mandate treatment with high-dose corticosteroids (prednisone, 60 mg daily) and prompt referral to a rheumatologist. Patients with ICI-associated PMR or GCA who require high-dose corticosteroids, or are unable to taper corticosteroids, can be treated with IL-6R blockade.[40] In milder cases, hydroxychloroquine or methotrexate can be used as a steroid-sparing agent.

Activated osteoarthritis

ICI-treated patients sometimes can present with severe pain in a single large joint, such as the hip or knee, and have evidence of osteoarthritis on radiographs of the affected joint. If synovial fluid analysis does not demonstrate inflammation, the authors refer to this painful condition as "activated osteoarthritis" (assuming metastatic disease and avascular necrosis have been ruled out). Most of these patients have had prior radiographs demonstrating osteoarthritis that predated treatment with ICI. With ICI treatment, however, they became more symptomatic or, less commonly, newly symptomatic. Painful flares of osteoarthritis in the non-ICI setting have been linked to inflammation at the microscopic level,[43] and it is likely that low-grade or subclinical inflammation is responsible for this ICI-associated phenomenon as well. Patients can be managed with NSAIDs and/or analgesics. Intraarticular injection of corticosteroids can be helpful. In cases of hip involvement, injections should be guided by ultrasound or fluoroscopy. Although the authors try to avoid systemic corticosteroids, at times a small dose of prednisone may be needed, especially if ICIs are continued. In cases of very advanced osteoarthritis, some patients may consider joint replacement, taking into consideration the prognosis of their malignancy.

Myositis

Myalgias (muscle pain) with or without CK elevation is reported in more than 20% of patients receiving nivolumab whereas true myositis, with muscle inflammation, weakness, and elevated CK occurs in less than 1% of patients who undergo therapy with a PD-1 inhibitor.[44] ICI-associated myositis often occurs early, within a month of ICI initiation.[45] Presentations can range from asymptomatic CK elevation to fulminant, diffuse weakness requiring ventilatory support. Although some patients present with proximal muscle weakness and elevated CK typical of de novo polymyositis, atypical muscle involvement also is described, including the of periorbital, bulbar, or paraspinal muscles, and CK sometimes can be severely elevated, up to 75 times the upper limit of normal, and associated with rhabdomyolysis.[46] Myositis-associated antibodies (such as antisynthetase antibodies) have been reported in some but not all series.[46,47] Patients with ICI myositis often have features of myasthenia gravis, such as diplopia and ptosis, although the results of electromyography (EMG), edrophonium (Tensilon) test, or cold pack testing not always are typical of those seen in de novo myasthenia.[45] Antistriated muscle antibodies commonly are seen in ICI myositis patients with features of myasthenia gravis, but antibodies to acetylcholine receptor are rarer. Patients with ICI myositis can have subtle (and not so subtle) concomitant myocarditis, and the converse also is true. According to a World Health Organization registry of myocarditis patients, 25% also had myositis.[48] ICI myocarditis is critical to identify because of its high case fatality rate, often due to arrhythmia. ICI myocarditis generally is associated with an elevated troponin I level, with or without changes on electrocardiography (EKG) or echocardiography.[49,50] Changes in EKG and/or echocardiography not always are present and cardiac MRI may be unremarkable, even in cases where endomyocardial biopsy shows inflammation.[19,51]

Muscle pathology in patients with ICI myositis demonstrates infiltration by histiocytes and cytotoxic T cells.[45] One autopsy study of 2 patients with ICI myositis demonstrated shared CD8+ T-cell clones in the tumor, heart, and skeletal muscle, suggesting the possibility of muscle injury due to cross-reactive T cells between the tumor and muscle.[52]

Treatment of ICI myositis depends on the severity of symptoms. Myalgia alone can be treated with NSAIDs or low-dose steroids, and ICI treatment does not need to be held unless there is severe pain and/or true muscle weakness. Patients with significant proximal weakness or any combination of the triad of myositis, myasthenia, and/or myocarditis require hospitalization and urgent treatment with high-dose corticosteroids. Some patients require intravenous immunoglobulin and/or plasmapheresis and immunosuppressive agents, such as mycophenolate mofetil.

Finally, although it can be difficult to distinguish ICI-induced myositis from a paraneoplastic inflammatory myositis clinically, the timing of myositis symptoms can help differentiation the 2—ICI myositis is likely to start within 1 month to 2 months of ICI treatment.[45–47] Dermatomyositis, which is more commonly paraneoplastic than polymyositis, is seen only rarely after ICI treatment.

Sicca disease

Sicca disease, or sicca syndrome, refers to dryness of the mouth and/or eyes due to exocrine gland dysfunction, symptoms that are typical of de novo Sjögren syndrome. ICI-associated sicca predominantly affects the mouth in contrast to non–ICI-related Sjögren, which results in dryness of both the eyes and mouth.[53] Sicca can follow treatment with both anti–PD-1/PD-L1 and anti–CTLA-4.[40,53] In clinical trials, the incidence of sicca in ICI-treated patients can be as high as 24%, although more often it affects 3% to 8% of treated patients.[40,54] Patients often report dry, cracked lips, difficulty chewing and swallowing food, altered taste, hoarseness, and difficulty swallowing food. When dryness affects the eyes, they often are described as gritty, with a sandlike sensation in the eye. Severe cases can lead to tongue fissuring and cavitation. It is important to rule out other causes of mouth irritation and pain, including pemphigoid (which also is seen in ICI-treated patients)[55] or concomitant chemotherapy causing stomatitis. Parotid swelling rarely is reported in ICI-treated patients, in contrast to de novo Sjögren syndrome. Occasionally, patients with ICI-associated sicca can have concomitant arthralgias but Sjögren antibodies (SSa/Ro and SSb/La) are present only rarely. Salivary gland histopathology demonstrates infiltration by T cells, and a notable absence of B cells, unlike de novo Sjögren, where infiltrating B cells predominate and germinal centers can be seen.[53]

Treatment of sicca depends on the severity of symptoms. Mild symptoms (grade 1, intermittently symptomatic without significant dietary alteration or visual disturbances) do not require the interruption of ICI therapy and can be treated with basic oral care, including good dental hygiene and the use of Biotene, an alcohol-free moisturizing mouthwash. Sugarless gum or sugar-free hard candy also can stimulate saliva production. Maintaining adequate hydration also is encouraged. Mild dry eye can be treated with over-the-counter refreshing eye drops. Moderate symptoms (grade 2, symptomatic with slightly altered oral intake and mild–moderate decrease in visual acuity) usually also do not require the interruption of ICI therapy and build on top of basic oral care with the addition of sialagogues, such as pilocarpine or cevimeline. Low-dose to moderate-dose corticosteroids may be required if symptoms persist. Severe symptoms (grade 3, interfering with ADLs, such as eating, speaking, and seeing) require cessation of ICI treatment and high-dose corticosteroids. Initial prednisone doses, of 20 mg per day to 40 mg per day for 2 weeks to 3 weeks, with a taper to follow, have shown favorable responses if treatment is started early.[53] Consultation with a dentist and/or ophthalmologist is recommended for patients with moderate or severe symptoms and when advanced therapies are needed, such as punctal plugs for severe dry eye. Although patients often improve symptomatically, salivary flow may not normalize.

Miscellaneous Rheumatic Disease

Sarcoid

Sarcoidosis or sarcoid-like reactions are not uncommon in ICI-treated individuals. Patients can present with rash or nodules, cough, arthralgias/arthritis, or inflammatory eye disease. Less commonly, granulomatous inflammation may be demonstrated in the spleen, bone marrow, or central nervous system.[56] Some patients are asymptomatic, however, and are diagnosed pathologically when noncaseating granulomas are found on biopsies done to evaluate changes on routine surveillance imaging, such as lymphadenopathy or pulmonary nodules. ICI sarcoid generally is steroid-responsive with steroid doses determined by the severity of symptoms, if there are any.[57] Treatment is not necessary in the absence of symptoms or other functionally significant changes. ICI sarcoid is not more common with anti–PD-1/PDL-1 or anti–CTLA-4 and there is no gender predisposition. Melanoma patients may be more likely to develop ICI sarcoid because they have an already higher incidence of sarcoidosis compared with the general population,[56] but melanoma patients also are the population most commonly treated with ICIs.

Vasculitis

Several case reports of vasculitis after ICI therapy have been described, including cutaneous leukocytoclastic vasculitis, eosinophilic granulomatosis with polyangiitis (formerly known as Churg-Strauss), granulomatosis with polyangiitis (formerly known as Wegener), GCA, and cryoglobulinemic vasculitis.[54] Typical symptoms of vasculitis, such as arthralgias or arthritis, palpable purpura, myalgias, fever, weight loss, and fatigue, have been described, although presentations vary. Although these manifestations have been described, vasculitis as an entity arising from ICI remains very rare. Serologies rarely are positive, so biopsy often is needed to establish a diagnosis.

Fibrosing skin disorders

Skin thickening has been reported as a rare rheumatic irAE, most commonly eosinophilic fasciitis rather than scleroderma. Eosinophilic fasciitis can result in severe joint contractures, pain, and muscle inflammation, and early recognition is important to minimize long-term morbidity.[58]

Systemic lupus erythematosus

Systemic lupus erythematosus (SLE) rarely is reported after ICI treatment, perhaps because ICI treatment is associated with high levels of interferon (IFN)-gamma rather than IFN-alpha, the putative driver of SLE. Subacute cutaneous lupus erythematosus has been described in a few ICI-treated patients presenting as the typical annular or psoriasiform eruption with an interface dermatitis on biopsy. Hydroxychloroquine and/or low-dose steroids can be used to treat these rare cases.

SUMMARY

In summary, there are a variety of rheumatic complications that can arise from treatment with ICI, with inflammatory arthritis and PMR the most common. ICI arthritis can affect quality of life significantly, and, although it usually can be treated rapidly and effectively, symptoms often persist and can require long-term treatment with corticosteroids and/or the addition of steroid-sparing agents. ICI myositis can have varying presentations from asymptomatic CK elevation to florid respiratory failure with diaphragmatic weakness as well as overlap symptoms with myocarditis and myasthenia gravis. Sicca symptoms after ICI vary in severity but at times require treatment with corticosteroids to prevent exocrine gland failure. SLE is extremely rare rheumatic after ICI, which may provide clues to the mechanism underlying irAEs.

CLINICS CARE POINTS

- When evaluating a patient with musculoskeletal pain, it is important to identify the affected organ—joint, muscle, nerve, or tendon.

- Joint pain after ICI can be inflammatory or mechanical and can be differentiated by the presence of swelling, morning stiffness greater than 30 minutes, and the pattern of joint distribution.

- PMR can be seen as a consequence of ICI therapy but may require higher doses of corticosteroids than are needed outside the ICI setting.

- Myositis often presents with myalgias, proximal muscle weakness, and elevated CK, but myasthenia-like bulbar and ocular involvement are common, as is concomitant myocarditis, and these overlap syndromes have a high fatality rate.

- Treatment of rheumatic irAEs always should be discussed with a patient's oncologist, and early rheumatology consultation usually is advisable.

DISCLOSURE

The authors have no commercial or financial conflicts of interest. N. Ghosh is supported by an NIH grant as a Master's degree student in Clinical and Translational Investigation at Weill Cornell Medicine: NIH/NCATS UL1-TR-0023849.

REFERENCES

1. Larkin J, Chiarion-Sileni V, Gonzalez R, et al. Combined Nivolumab and Ipilimumab or Monotherapy in Untreated Melanoma. N Engl J Med 2015;373(1):23–34.
2. Ribas A, Wolchok JD. Cancer immunotherapy using checkpoint blockade. Science 2018;359(6382):1350–5.

3. Topalian SL, Drake CG, Pardoll DM. Immune checkpoint blockade: a common denominator approach to cancer therapy. Cancer Cell 2015;27(4):450–61.

4. Marcus L, Lemery SJ, Keegan P, et al. FDA Approval Summary: Pembrolizumab for the Treatment of Microsatellite Instability-High Solid Tumors. Clin Cancer Res 2019;25(13):3753–8.

5. Overman MJ, Lonardi S, Wong KYM, et al. Durable Clinical Benefit With Nivolumab Plus Ipilimumab in DNA Mismatch Repair-Deficient/Microsatellite Instability-High Metastatic Colorectal Cancer. J Clin Oncol 2018;36(8):773–9.

6. Chan KK, Bass AR. Autoimmune complications of immunotherapy: pathophysiology and management. BMJ 2020;369:m736.

7. Postow MA, Sidlow R, Hellmann MD. Immune-Related Adverse Events Associated with Immune Checkpoint Blockade. N Engl J Med 2018;378(2):158–68.

8. Arnaud-Coffin P, Maillet D, Gan HK, et al. A systematic review of adverse events in randomized trials assessing immune checkpoint inhibitors. Int J Cancer 2019; 145(3):639–48.

9. Common Terminology Criteria for Adverse Events (CTCAE) Version 5.0. 2017. Available at: https://ctep.cancer.gov/protocoldevelopment/electronic_applications/docs/CTCAE_v5_Quick_Reference_8.5x11.pdf. Accessed June 18, 2020.

10. Sznol M, Ferrucci PF, Hogg D, et al. Pooled Analysis Safety Profile of Nivolumab and Ipilimumab Combination Therapy in Patients With Advanced Melanoma. J Clin Oncol 2017;35(34):3815–22.

11. Weber JS, Hodi FS, Wolchok JD, et al. Safety Profile of Nivolumab Monotherapy: A Pooled Analysis of Patients With Advanced Melanoma. J Clin Oncol 2017;35(7):785–92.

12. Wang DY, Salem JE, Cohen JV, et al. Fatal Toxic Effects Associated With Immune Checkpoint Inhibitors: A Systematic Review and Meta-analysis. JAMA Oncol 2018;4(12):1721–8.

13. Zhou X, Yao Z, Yang H, et al. Are immune-related adverse events associated with the efficacy of immune checkpoint inhibitors in patients with cancer? A systematic review and meta-analysis. BMC Med 2020;18(1):87.

14. Freeman-Keller M, Kim Y, Cronin H, et al. Nivolumab in Resected and Unresectable Metastatic Melanoma: Characteristics of Immune-Related Adverse Events and Association with Outcomes. Clin Cancer Res 2016;22(4):886–94.

15. Teulings HE, Limpens J, Jansen SN, et al. Vitiligo-like depigmentation in patients with stage III-IV melanoma receiving immunotherapy and its association with survival: a systematic review and meta-analysis. J Clin Oncol 2015;33(7):773–81.

16. Maher VE, Fernandes LL, Weinstock C, et al. Analysis of the Association Between Adverse Events and Outcome in Patients Receiving a Programmed Death Protein 1 or Programmed Death Ligand 1 Antibody. J Clin Oncol 2019;37(30):2730–7.

17. Salem JE, Allenbach Y, Vozy A, et al. Abatacept for Severe Immune Checkpoint Inhibitor-Associated Myocarditis. N Engl J Med 2019;380(24):2377–9.

18. Abdel-Wahab N, Shah M, Lopez-Olivo MA, et al. Use of Immune Checkpoint Inhibitors in the Treatment of Patients With Cancer and Preexisting Autoimmune Disease: A Systematic Review. Ann Intern Med 2018;168(2):121–30.

19. Leung AM, Farewell D, Lau CS, et al. Defining criteria for rheumatoid arthritis patient-derived disease activity score that correspond to Disease Activity Score 28 and Clinical Disease Activity Index based disease states and response criteria. Rheumatology (Oxford) 2016;55(11):1954–8.

20. Abu-Sbeih H, Ali FS, Wang X, et al. Early introduction of selective immunosuppressive therapy associated with favorable clinical outcomes in patients with immune checkpoint inhibitor–induced colitis. J Immunother Cancer 2019;7(1):93.

21. Johnson DH, Zobniw CM, Trinh VA, et al. Infliximab associated with faster symptom resolution compared with corticosteroids alone for the management of immune-related enterocolitis. J Immunother Cancer 2018;6(1):103.

22. Wang Y, Abu-Sbeih H, Mao E, et al. Immune-checkpoint inhibitor-induced diarrhea and colitis in patients with advanced malignancies: retrospective review at MD Anderson. J Immunother Cancer 2018;6(1):37.

23. Cappelli LC, Brahmer JR, Forde PM, et al. Clinical presentation of immune checkpoint inhibitor-induced inflammatory arthritis differs by immunotherapy regimen. Semin Arthritis Rheum 2018;48(3):553–7.

24. Smith MH, Bass AR. Arthritis after cancer immunotherapy: symptom duration and treatment response. Arthritis Care Res 2019;71(3):362–6.

25. Faje AT, Lawrence D, Flaherty K, et al. High-dose glucocorticoids for the treatment of ipilimumab-induced hypophysitis is associated with reduced survival in patients with melanoma. Cancer 2018;124(18):3706–14.

26. Verheijden RJ, May AM, Blank CU, et al. Association of Anti-TNF with Decreased Survival in Steroid Refractory Ipilimumab and Anti-PD1-Treated Patients in the Dutch Melanoma Treatment Registry. Clin Cancer Res 2020;26(9):2268–74.

27. Braaten TJ, Brahmer JR, Forde PM, et al. Immune checkpoint inhibitor-induced inflammatory arthritis persists after immunotherapy cessation. Ann Rheum Dis 2020;79(3):332–8.

28. Perez-Ruiz E, Minute L, Otano I, et al. Prophylactic TNF blockade uncouples efficacy and toxicity in dual CTLA-4 and PD-1 immunotherapy. Nature 2019;569(7756): 428–32.

29. Kostine M, Rouxel L, Barnetche T, et al. Rheumatic disorders associated with immune checkpoint inhibitors in patients with cancer—clinical aspects and relationship with tumour response: a single-centre prospective cohort study. Ann Rheum Dis 2018;77(3):393–8.

30. Ghosh N, Tiongson MD, Stewart C, et al. Checkpoint Inhibitor-Associated Arthritis: A Systematic Review of Case Reports and Case Series. J Clin Rheumatol 2020. https://doi.org/10.1097/RHU.0000000000001370. Epub ahead of print. PMID: 32345841.

31. Richter MD, Crowson C, Kottschade LA, et al. Rheumatic Syndromes Associated With Immune Checkpoint Inhibitors: A Single-Center Cohort of Sixty-One Patients. Arthritis Rheum 2019;71(3):468–75.

32. Leipe J, Christ LA, Arnoldi AP, et al. Characteristics and treatment of new-onset arthritis after checkpoint inhibitor therapy. RMD Open 2018;4(2):e000714.

33. de Moel EC, Rozeman EA, Kapiteijn EHW, et al. Autoantibody development under treatment with immune checkpoint inhibitors. Cancer Immunol Res 2019;7(1):6–11.

34. Gregersen PK, Silver J, Winchester RJ. The shared epitope hypothesis. An approach to understanding the molecular genetics of susceptibility to rheumatoid arthritis. Arthritis Rheum 1987;30(11):1205–13.

35. Klareskog L, Stolt P, Lundberg K, et al. A new model for an etiology of rheumatoid arthritis: smoking may trigger HLA-DR (shared epitope)-restricted immune reactions to autoantigens modified by citrullination. Arthritis Rheum 2006;54(1):38–46.

36. Cappelli LC, Dorak MT, Bettinotti MP, et al. Association of HLA-DRB1 shared epitope alleles and immune checkpoint inhibitor-induced inflammatory arthritis. Rheumatology (Oxford) 2019;58(3):476–80.

37. Guo Y, Walsh AM, Canavan M, et al. Immune checkpoint inhibitor PD-1 pathway is down-regulated in synovium at various stages of rheumatoid arthritis disease progression. PLoS One 2018;13(2):e0192704.

428   Ghosh & Bass

38. Roberts J, Smylie M, Walker J, et al. Hydroxychloroquine is a safe and effective steroid-sparing agent for immune checkpoint inhibitor–induced inflammatory arthritis. Clin Rheumatol 2019;38(5):1513–9.
39. Kim ST, Tayar J, Suarez-Almazor M, et al. Successful treatment of arthritis induced by checkpoint inhibitors with tocilizumab: a case series. Ann Rheum Dis 2017;76(12):2061–4.
40. Calabrese C, Cappelli LC, Kostine M, et al. Polymyalgia rheumatica-like syndrome from checkpoint inhibitor therapy: case series and systematic review of the literature. RMD Open 2019;5(1):e000906.
41. Betrains A, Blockmans DE. Immune Checkpoint Inhibitor-Associated Polymyalgia Rheumatica/Giant Cell Arteritis Occurring in a Patient After Treatment With Nivolumab. J Clin Rheumatol 2019. https://doi.org/10.1097/RHU.0000000000001012. Epub ahead of print. PMID: 30801332.
42. Micaily I, Chernoff M. An unknown reaction to pembrolizumab: giant cell arteritis. Ann Oncol 2017;28(10):2621–2.
43. Scanzello CR. Role of low-grade inflammation in osteoarthritis. Curr Opin Rheumatol 2017;29(1):79–85.
44. <pi_opdivo.pdf>. In: Squibb B-M, editor. packageinserts. Available at: packageinserts.bms.com/pi/pi_opdivo.pdf. Accessed October 23, 2020.
45. Seki M, Uruha A, Ohnuki Y, et al. Inflammatory myopathy associated with PD-1 inhibitors. J Autoimmun 2019;100:105–13.
46. Shah M, Tayar JH, Abdel-Wahab N, et al. Myositis as an adverse event of immune checkpoint blockade for cancer therapy. Semin Arthritis Rheum 2019;48(4):736–40.
47. Moreira A, Loquai C, Pföhler C, et al. Myositis and neuromuscular side-effects induced by immune checkpoint inhibitors. Eur J Cancer 2019;106:12–23.
48. Moslehi JJ, Salem JE, Sosman JA, et al. Increased reporting of fatal immune checkpoint inhibitor-associated myocarditis. Lancet 2018;391(10124):933.
49. Ganatra S, Neilan TG. Immune Checkpoint Inhibitor-Associated Myocarditis. Oncologist 2018;23(8):879–86.
50. Mahmoud F, Wilkinson JT, Gizinski A, et al. Could knee inflammatory synovitis be induced by pembrolizumab? J Oncol Pharm Pract 2018;24(5):389–92.
51. Escudier M, Cautela J, Malissen N, et al. Clinical Features, Management, and Outcomes of Immune Checkpoint Inhibitor-Related Cardiotoxicity. Circulation 2017;136(21):2085–7.
52. Johnson DB, Balko JM, Compton ML, et al. Fulminant Myocarditis with Combination Immune Checkpoint Blockade. N Engl J Med 2016;375(18):1749–55.
53. Warner BM, Baer AN, Lipson EJ, et al. Sicca Syndrome Associated with Immune Checkpoint Inhibitor Therapy. Oncologist 2019;24(9):1259–69.
54. Cappelli LC, Gutierrez AK, Bingham CO III, et al. Rheumatic and musculoskeletal immune-related adverse events due to immune checkpoint inhibitors: a systematic review of the literature. Arthritis Care Res 2017;69(11):1751–63.
55. Naidoo J, Schindler K, Querfeld C, et al. Autoimmune Bullous Skin Disorders with Immune Checkpoint Inhibitors Targeting PD-1 and PD-L1. Cancer Immunol Res 2016;4(5):383–9.
56. Rambhia PH, Reichert B, Scott JF, et al. Immune checkpoint inhibitor-induced sarcoidosis-like granulomas. Int J Clin Oncol 2019;24(10):1171–81.
57. Gkiozos I, Kopitopoulou A, Kalkanis A, et al. Sarcoidosis-Like Reactions Induced by Checkpoint Inhibitors. J Thorac Oncol 2018;13(8):1076–82.
58. Chan KK, Magro C, Shoushtari A, et al. Eosinophilic Fasciitis Following Checkpoint Inhibitor Therapy: Four Cases and a Review of Literature. Oncologist 2020;25(2):140–9.

Managing Cardiovascular Risk in Patients with Rheumatic Disease

Lyn D. Ferguson, MBChB(Hons), PhD, MRCP(UK)[a],[*],
Naveed Sattar, MBChB, PhD, FRCP[a], Iain B. McInnes, MBChB, PhD, FRCP[b]

KEYWORDS

- RA • SLE • Gout • Cardiovascular disease (CVD) • Inflammation

KEY POINTS

- Rheumatoid arthritis, gout, and systemic lupus erythematosus are associated with increased cardiovascular disease (CVD) risk compared with the general population.
- This risk is related to a combination of traditional cardiovascular risk factors, disease-specific factors, and some medications including NSAIDs and prolonged use of relatively high-dose corticosteroids.
- CVD risk should be assessed using relevant national or international risk assessment tools. These may need to be adapted in RMDs with a multiplication factor.
- Management includes lifestyle modifications and pharmacological treatment of traditional cardiovascular risk factors, as well as tight control of disease activity with disease-modifying-antirheumatic drugs.
- Nonsteroidal anti-inflammatory drugs should be used with caution. Corticosteroids should be prescribed at the lowest effective dose for the shortest possible duration.

INTRODUCTION

Individuals with chronic inflammatory rheumatic and musculoskeletal diseases (RMDs), notably rheumatoid arthritis (RA), systemic lupus erythematosus (SLE), and gout, are at increased risk of cardiovascular disease (CVD) compared with the general population. Central to all 3 conditions is chronic inflammation. Many of the cellular and molecular features of RMDs now also are recognized as operant in the pathogenesis of CVD, especially in the local lesions of atherosclerosis and in promoting wider endothelial

This article originally appeared in the Medical Clinics of North America, Volume 105, Issue 2, March 2021.

[a] Institute of Cardiovascular and Medical Sciences, University of Glasgow, 126 University Place, Glasgow G12 8TA, UK; [b] Institute of Infection, Immunity and Inflammation, University of Glasgow, 126 University Place, Glasgow G12 8TA, UK

* Corresponding author. Institute of Cardiovascular and Medical Sciences, BHF GCRC, University of Glasgow, Room 213, 126 University Place, Glasgow G12 8TA, UK.

E-mail address: Lyn.Ferguson@glasgow.ac.uk

and microvascular dysfunction. The combination of RMD-specific factors coupled with a higher prevalence of traditional cardiovascular risk factors, for example, smoking, hypertension, dyslipidemia, diabetes, and obesity, and certain medications, for example, several nonsteroidal anti-inflammatory drugs (NSAIDs), the cyclooxygenase (COX)-2 inhibitor rofecoxib, and prolonged use of relatively high dose corticosteroids, all contribute to greater CVD morbidity and mortality in chronic RMDs (**Fig. 1**).

In this article, the authors review the evidence base for CVD risk in RA, SLE, and gout, drawn largely from observational studies, and consider potential mechanisms for such increased risk. Then how best to manage cardiovascular risk in chronic RMDs is discussed by addressing traditional risk factors through lifestyle and pharmacotherapy as well as treating underlying systemic inflammation through antirheumatic therapies.

DISCUSSION
Cardiovascular Disease Risk in Rheumatoid Arthritis

RA is associated with increased CVD risk. Previous meta-analysis has shown those with RA have a 48% higher risk of incident CVD, 68% higher risk of myocardial infarction (MI), and 41% higher risk of stroke compared with the general population.[1] More recent estimates suggest this excess risk may be less than previously estimated, with data from the QResearch database in the United Kingdom suggesting around a 24% greater CVD risk in RA compared with the general population.[2] Although this may relate to better treatments now available for RA, individuals with RA remain at greater cardiovascular risk than their non-RA counterparts, likely related to a combination of a higher prevalence of traditional cardiovascular risk factors, for example, smoking,

RMD specific factors: **Traditional CVD risk factors:**

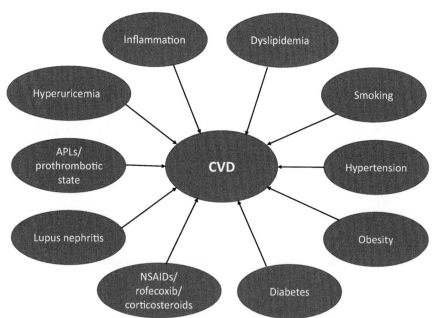

Fig. 1. A combination of traditional cardiovascular risk factors, disease-specific factors, and some commonly prescribed medications, including certain NSAIDs, the COX-2 inhibitor rofecoxib, and corticosteroids (dose and duration dependent), contribute to increased CVD risk in RMDs.

obesity, physical inactivity, hyperlipidemia, type 2 diabetes mellitus, and hypertension as well as underlying chronic inflammation.[3] A large international study, A Trans-Atlantic Cardiovascular Consortium for Rheumatoid Arthritis, revealed approximately 49% of CVD events in RA were attributable to traditional CVD risk factors (in particular, smoking and hypertension) and 30% to RA characteristics (elevated DAS28, rheumatoid factor/anti-citrullinated protein antibody positive, and raised erythrocyte sedimentation rate and C-reactive protein [CRP]).[4] Cardiovascular mortality also is increased in RA, in the order of 43% to 66% higher than the general population, even after adjustment for age, sex, and traditional cardiovascular risk factors.[5]

Traditional cardiovascular risk factors

Prior meta-analysis of RA patients revealed those with concomitant hypertension and diabetes were at 84% and 89% higher risk of MI, respectively, compared with those without these risk factors.[6] CVD morbidity in RA was greater in those with hypertension (relative risk [RR] 2.24), type 2 diabetes mellitus (RR 1.94), smoking (RR 1.50), hypercholesterolemia (RR 1.73) ,and obesity (RR 1.16),[6] highlighting the important contribution of traditional cardiovascular risk factors to overall CVD risk in RA.

Although dyslipidemia, in particular, elevated low-density lipoprotein (LDL) cholesterol, is strongly associated with increased CVD risk in the general population, its role in RA is more complicated. Those with RA may display an apparent lipid paradox, with reduced total cholesterol and LDL cholesterol, despite RA being an independent risk factor for CVD.[7] This may relate to the state of active inflammation in RA with activation of the mononuclear phagocyte system that scavenges LDL particles, resulting in lowered serum LDL cholesterol concentrations.[8] Subsequent treatment to reduce inflammation generally leads to a rise in serum LDL cholesterol concentrations,[9] especially apparent with the interleukin (IL)-6 receptor antagonist tocilizumab[10] and is thought to be linked to a reversal of IL-6–induced LDL cholesterol clearance from the circulation.[8] Similar patterns of lipid changes have been observed across studies of Janus kinase inhibitors, which inhibit signaling downstream of IL-6.[11,12] For example, treatment with tofacitinib resulted in reduced clearance of LDL cholesterol particles from the circulation and an increase in circulating cholesterol concentrations.[13]

An obesity paradox also may exist in RA with an inverse relationship between body mass index (BMI) and mortality. Although increased BMI is associated with CVD mortality in the general population,[14] in contrast, individuals with RA who are overweight or obese appear to have a lower RR of all-cause and CVD mortality than patients with a normal BMI (18.5–24.9 kg/m²).[15] Importantly, a separate study demonstrated this inverse association between BMI and mortality was lost after adjustment for comorbidities and RA severity.[16] This suggests the obesity paradox of RA may be due to residual confounding and reverse causality whereby active inflammatory disease leads to unintentional weight loss.[17] Supporting this, evidence has shown weight loss, rather than current BMI, is a strong predictor of mortality in RA, with a fall in BMI of greater than or equal to1 kg/m² associated with almost twice the risk of death.[18]

Rheumatoid arthritis disease-specific factors

Although traditional cardiovascular risk factors significantly contribute to CVD risk in RA, disease-specific factors also play an important role. Studies have demonstrated an association between higher cumulative inflammatory burden and increased CVD risk in RA.[19–23] Although disease duration does not appear to affect CVD risk independently,[20] disease activity as well as the number and duration of flares over time may contribute to greater CVD risk in RA.[19–22]

The heightened state of chronic inflammation has long been hypothesized to contribute to increased CVD risk in RA. Both RA and atherosclerosis share similar underlying inflammatory pathways. These comprise T-cell and myeloid lineage cell activation, release of proinflammatory cytokines, and increased leukocyte adhesion molecule expression.[24] Inflamed synovium in affected joints as well as secondary lymphoid tissues, including the spleen, lymph nodes, and adipose tissue, release proinflammatory cytokines, such as tumor necrosis factor (TNF), IL-1β, IL-6, and immune complexes into the circulation. Complement activation also is a feature. This in turn can have numerous systemic adverse effects on skeletal muscle, liver, vascular tissue, adipose tissue, and circulating lipid profiles, leading to insulin resistance, increased CRP and procoagulant production from the liver, endothelial dysfunction, increased arterial stiffness, atherosclerotic plaque formation, and potentially altered body composition with increased central abdominal fat and decreased lean mass. Collectively, these changes may culminate in CVD.[25]

Individuals with RA have been shown to have increased arterial wall inflammation on fluorodeoxyglucose PET/computed tomography imaging, which attenuated with anti-TNF therapy.[26] Furthermore, RA is associated with greater atherosclerotic burden, including increased carotid intima-media thickness, carotid plaque burden,[27] and coronary plaques,[28] in particular noncalcified and mixed plaques, which appear more vulnerable to rupture than fully calcified plaques.[28,29]

Medications

Some medications commonly used to treat RA, namely certain NSAIDs, in particular diclofenac, and the now withdrawn COX-2 inhibitor rofecoxib, as well as the prolonged use of relatively high-dose corticosteroids, also contribute to increased CVD risk in RA.[30] Their association is discussed in further detail later.

Summary

CVD risk is increased in RA and is related to a combination of traditional cardiovascular risk factors; disease-specific factors, namely chronic inflammation; and some commonly prescribed medications, including certain NSAIDs as well as prolonged courses of relatively high-dose corticosteroids.

Cardiovascular Disease Risk in Gout

In contrast to RA, studies examining the association between gout and incident coronary heart disease (CHD) have been more mixed. Two studies, The Meharry-Hopkins study[31] and a separate Dutch primary care study by Janssens and colleagues,[32] did not show a significant independent association of gout with CVD. In contrast, a study of more than 5000 individuals from the Framingham Heart Study demonstrated men with gout had a 60% excess risk of CHD compared with men without gout.[33] This excess risk was related in part to a greater prevalence of traditional cardiovascular risk factors, for example, hypertension, hypercholesterolemia, alcohol, and elevated BMI. Even after adjustment for these risk factors, however, excess CHD risk remained. The reasons for such disparities between studies may relate to differences in underlying study populations, design, and sample size.

A separate study of more than 51,000 men in the Health Professionals Follow-Up Study reaffirmed an independent association of gout with all-cause and CVD mortality.[34] After adjusting for traditional risk factors, men with gout (without prior CHD) had a 28% higher all-cause mortality, 38% higher CVD mortality, and 55% higher CHD mortality compared with men without gout. Similarly, data from the Multiple Risk

Factor Intervention Trial (MRFIT) of more than 12,000 men revealed gout was associated with a 26% higher risk of acute MI after adjustment for known cardiovascular risk factors.

Despite the earlier Framingham study demonstrating no association between gout and CHD in women, a later primary care study using the UK Clinical Practice Research Datalink demonstrated female patients with gout were at greatest risk of incident vascular events, even after adjustment for vascular risk factors, despite a higher prevalence of both gout and vascular disease in men.[35] The reason for such sex differences in vascular risk remain to be fully determined but may include more prolonged exposure to hyperuricemia in women, who generally require a higher mean serum uric acid level to develop gout.[36] Decreasing estrogen during the menopause also may have a detrimental effect on renal uric acid excretion[37] and contribute to increased central (abdominal) obesity associated with increased cardiometabolic risk.[38] Finally, it is possible clinicians may be less vigilant in prompt diagnosis and treatment of gout and CVD in women due to the male preponderance of these conditions.

Potential mechanisms

Central to gout pathogenesis is hyperuricemia with urate crystal deposition in joints. Beyond acute joint inflammation, elevated serum urate levels have been associated with increased CHD incidence and mortality.[39] This may relate in part to the association of hyperuricemia with traditional risk factors, including hypertension, dyslipidemia, chronic kidney disease, and overweight/obesity.[40]

Hyperuricemia is closely associated with endothelial dysfunction, an early marker of atherosclerosis.[41,42] In a study of 46 hyperuricemic patients matched with 46 age-matched and sex-matched healthy controls, hyperuricemic individuals had significantly lower flow-mediated dilation values than controls, indicative of worse endothelial function.[43] In a later study of postmenopausal women who underwent coronary microvascular function testing to assess for coronary endothelial dysfunction (CED), individuals with CED had significantly higher uric acid levels compared with those without CED.[44]

Elevated serum urate levels have been associated with greater smooth- cell proliferation, LDL oxidation, and platelet activation as well as a potential role in hypertension pathogenesis, suggesting an etiologic role for hyperuricemia in atherosclerotic disease.[45] It also is possible, however, that hyperuricemia simply may represent a surrogate marker for high levels of damaging oxidative stress associated with increased xanthine oxidase activity rather than being directly responsible for vascular injury per se.[45]

A further potential mechanistic link between hyperuricemia and CVD may include activation of the NLRP3 inflammasome by monosodium urate crystals. This may contribute to increased CVD through the release of IL-1β.[46] Inhibition of IL-1β receptor binding with canakinumab, used clinically to treat gout, has been shown to reduce recurrent vascular events in the Canakinumab Anti-inflammatory Thrombosis Outcome Study (CANTOS).[47]

Summary

Although some studies have been conflicting, there now is increasing evidence that gout is associated with increased CVD risk. This is related to both a greater prevalence of traditional cardiovascular risk factors, including hypertension, hypercholesterolemia, alcohol, and elevated BMI, and underlying hyperuricemia and systemic inflammation.

Cardiovascular Disease Risk in Systemic Lupus Erythematosus

SLE, a multisystem autoimmune disease affecting primarily women of childbearing age, is associated with significantly greater cardiovascular risk. Although the exact frequency of cardiovascular events in SLE varies, an early study from the University of Pittsburgh Medical Center found approximately 7% of SLE patients had a cardiovascular event, with patients in the 35-year-old to 44-year-old age group more than 50 times more likely to have an MI than those without SLE.[48] Factors associated with greater CVD risk included an older age at lupus diagnosis, longer disease duration, longer duration of corticosteroid use, hypercholesterolemia, and being postmenopausal.[48]

Despite improvements in disease management, a more contemporary study of individuals from the UK Biobank demonstrated SLE still is associated with significant cardiometabolic risk.[49] SLE participants displayed several traditional risk factors, including hypertension, hypercholesterolemia, obesity, and smoking. After adjustment for age, gender, ethnicity, deprivation index, educational level, antihypertensive medications, and lipid-lowering medications, SLE was associated with an almost 3-fold greater risk of CHD, a more than 4-fold greater risk of stroke, a more than 5-fold greater risk of VTE, and a more than 15-fold greater risk of PAD.[49] Longer disease duration as well as NSAID/corticosteroid use were associated with greater cardiometabolic risk.[49]

Corticosteroids are known to be associated with increased CVD risk in the general population, in the order of 58% to 81% for men and women, respectively, compared with those not taking corticosteroid medications.[2] Even after adjusting for corticosteroid use, however, as well as traditional cardiovascular risk factors, data from The QResearch database showed women with SLE still had more than double the risk of developing CVD, and men with SLE approximately 55% greater CVD risk compared with the general population.[2]

Potential mechanisms

In addition to traditional risk factors and NSAID/corticosteroid use, several SLE-specific factors may contribute to heightened CVD risk in this group. Chronic damage, as assessed by the Systemic Lupus International Collaborating Clinics damage index, was found to be independently associated with increased carotid intima-media thickness scores, carotid plaque formation, and arterial stiffness.[50–52] The presence of lupus nephritis also was associated with greater odds of carotid plaque compared with age-matched non-nephritis SLE patients and population controls.[53] Certain genetic variants, such as those in the risk allele for SLE in the signal transducer and activator of transcription factor 4 (STAT4) gene, also have been associated with vascular events, in particular, ischemic cerebrovascular disease.[54]

Although the exact mechanisms underlying atherosclerosis in SLE remain to be determined, it is thought there is an imbalance between endothelial damage and atheroprotective mechanisms.[55] Damage to the endothelium may result from deposition of oxidized LDL and previous data have shown higher levels of oxidized epitopes on LDL in SLE patients compared with age-matched and sex-matched controls.[56] Several autoantibodies, including antiendothelial cell antibodies and antiphospholipid antibodies (APLs), may contribute to endothelial injury in SLE.[55] APLs also contribute to a prothrombotic state.[57] Type 1 interferons, involved in the pathogenesis of SLE, may promote premature vascular damage in SLE.[58] Neutrophil extracellular traps also may play a role in SLE-related atherosclerosis because they are thought to be prothrombotic and may impair antiatherogenic HDL.[59] Immune complexes also may play a role in atherosclerotic lesion development.[60] Finally, impaired atheroprotective mechanisms, including impaired endothelial repair and decreased production of atheroprotective autoantibodies, also may contribute.

Summary

In summary, SLE is associated with significantly increased CVD risk. This is related to a combination of traditional cardiovascular risk factors, NSAID/corticosteroid use, and disease-specific factors, including accumulating chronic disease damage, lupus nephritis, genetic factors, prothrombotic APLs, and imbalances between endothelial damage and atheroprotective mechanisms.

Managing Cardiovascular Disease Risk in Rheumatic Diseases

There are 2 main approaches to targeting the increased CVD risk associated with chronic RMDs. These include targeting traditional CVD risk factors through lifestyle and pharmacologic interventions and tight control of underlying disease activity.

Traditional cardiovascular disease risk factors

Individuals with RMDs should be screened for traditional cardiovascular risk factors and their total cardiovascular risk assessed with the aid of a CVD risk prediction model. It is recognized that several of the risk prediction models designed for the general population, for example, the Systematic Coronary Risk Evaluation (SCORE) and Framingham risk score, may underestimate future CVD risk in individuals with RA because they do not include nontraditional risk factors.[61,62] At present, however, there are no alternative CVD risk prediction models with proven accuracy and superiority in inflammatory joint diseases. In an attempt to address this issue, current European League Against Rheumatism (EULAR) guidelines recommend CVD risk prediction models should be adapted for patients with RA by a 1.5 multiplication factor (if this is not already included in the risk algorithm).[63]

As in the general population, lifestyle interventions, including smoking cessation and regular physical activity, are important to lower CVD risk in inflammatory joint disease. Studies have shown exercise has several cardiovascular benefits in RA, improving cardiorespiratory fitness and microvascular and macrovascular function and decreasing cardiovascular risk.[64,65]

In addition to lifestyle interventions, management of hypertension and dyslipidemia with antihypertensive and lipid-lowering therapies also is important. Data from the general population show a 10–mm Hg reduction in systolic blood pressure is associated with a 20% reduction in CVD events,[66] and a 1-mmol/L reduction in LDL cholesterol with statin therapy is associated with an approximately 20% reduction in major adverse cardiovascular events (MACEs).[67] The benefit of statin therapy in CVD risk reduction in RA recently was demonstrated in the Trial of Atorvastatin for the Primary Prevention of Cardiovascular Events in Patients with Rheumatoid Arthritis.[68] This randomized placebo-controlled trial showed individuals with RA prescribed atorvastatin, 40 mg, had a mean ($\pm$SD) reduction in LDL cholesterol of 0.77 ($\pm$0.04) mmol/L compared with placebo ($P<.0001$). Of the 1504 patients receiving atorvastatin, 24 (1.6%) experienced the primary composite cardiovascular endpoint compared with 36 (2.4%) of the 1498 receiving placebo (hazard ratio [HR] 0.66; 95% CI, 0.39, 1.11; $P = 0.115$). Although this reduction was not statistically significant, likely related to the study having a lower than expected event rate, the reduction in CVD risk with the given reduction in LDL cholesterol concentration was consistent with the Cholesterol Treatment Trialists' Collaboration meta-analysis of statin effects in other populations. There also were no significant differences in adverse event rates between statin and placebo, showing atorvastatin, 40 mg, was safe in the setting of RA.[68]

Antirheumatic therapies

Inflammation is central to RA, gout, SLE, and atherosclerosis pathogenesis. Consequently, antirheumatic therapies that lower inflammation should lower cardiovascular risk, although this relationship may vary according to the medication chosen. The following sections outline the effects of current antirheumatic therapies on CVD risk in inflammatory rheumatic diseases.

Nonsteroidal anti-inflammatory drugs and cyclooxygenase 2 inhibitors Several nonselective NSAIDs, as well as the selective COX-2 inhibitor rofecoxib, have been associated with increased CVD risk, although this relationship may vary according to the individual medication chosen.[30] For example, studies have shown diclofenac and the selective COX-2 inhibitor rofecoxib were associated with increased risk of MI and CHD death, particularly at higher doses.[69–71] Rofecoxib was withdrawn in 2004 when it was demonstrated to be associated with almost twice the risk of cardiovascular thrombotic events compared with placebo treatment.[72] On the other hand, moderate doses of the COX-2 inhibitor celecoxib were found to be noninferior to ibuprofen or naproxen with regard to cardiovascular safety, noting the limitations of a noninferiority study.[73] A large, well-conducted meta-analysis of trial data found that treatment with naproxen resulted in no excess risk of major cardiovascular events (RR 0.93; 95% CI, 0.69–1.27).[70]

Corticosteroids Although corticosteroids are effective at dampening inflammation in inflammatory joint disease, these drugs have notable long-term effects on morbidity and mortality. A large general population study demonstrated women and men prescribed long-term oral corticosteroids had 82% and 58% higher cardiovascular risk, respectively, compared with those not prescribed corticosteroid therapy.[2] The adverse effects of corticosteroids in RA have been shown to be dose and duration dependent, with relatively high daily prednisone doses (starting from 8 mg/day to 15 mg/day), a high cumulative dose, and a longer exposure to corticosteroids (in years) associated with greater CVD risk.[74] Other studies also have shown increased risk of type 2 diabetes mellitus, hypertension, thrombotic stroke or MI, and death with corticosteroid use.[75,76]

Despite these findings, some argue that in patients with active RA, the anti-inflammatory benefits of corticosteroids potentially may counteract some of these detrimental CVD effects, and a study, the Glucocorticoid Low-dose Outcome in Rheumatoid Arthritis Study, currently is under way to address this issue.[77] For the meantime, however, it generally is advised that clinicians should prescribe the lowest dose of glucocorticoids for the shortest time possible.

Conventional synthetic disease-modifying antirheumatic drugs Methotrexate has been associated with reduced all-cause and CVD mortality in individuals with RA.[78] Meta-analysis revealed methotrexate was associated with a 21% lower risk of total CVD and an 18% lower risk of MI in patients with RA, psoriasis, or polyarthritis.[79] These observational findings suggest that methotrexate may reduce cardiovascular risk in inflammatory joint disease through targeting inflammation. In the Cardiovascular Inflammation Reduction Trial (CIRT), treatment with low-dose methotrexate did not reduce the rate of cardiovascular events in patients with established CVD,[80] leading some to question whether methotrexate is cardioprotective. Mean serum CRP concentrations, however, in CIRT participants were substantially lower than those typically found in RA.

Conventional synthetic DMARDs also may have metabolic effects, including altering body composition and the risk of diabetes. For example, treatment with either methotrexate, prednisone, or a TNF inhibitor may be associated with weight gain, whereas leflunomide is associated with modest weight loss in RA. In observational studies of patients with RA, patients taking hydroxychloroquine or abatacept were less likely to develop diabetes, whereas those taking glucocorticoids were more likely to develop diabetes, compared with patients prescribed methotrexate monotherapy.[81,82]

Biologic therapies Anti-TNF therapy is effective at lowering inflammation and improving disease activity in RA.[83] Because systemic inflammation is thought to drive cardiovascular risk, it follows TNF inhibition should lower this risk. In an observational study of patients with RA, although the rate of MI was similar in patients taking a TNF inhibitor to those taking conventional synthetic DMARDs, those who clinically responded to anti-TNF therapy demonstrated a 64% lower rate of MI compared with nonresponders.[84] Meta-analyses subsequently have shown TNF inhibitors were associated with significant reductions in the risk of all cardiovascular events (RR, 0.70; 95% CI, 0.54–0.90; $P = 0.005$), including MI, stroke, and major adverse cardiac events.[30,85]

Although TNF inhibitors may have beneficial effects on decreasing CVD risk, other biologics, notably the IL-6 inhibitor tocilizumab and the JAK-inhibitor tofacitinib, have been associated with an increase in total cholesterol and LDL cholesterol concentrations.[10,13] This effect simply may be part of a compensatory response to dampened inflammation, but the long-term cardiovascular sequelae of these lipid alterations remain to be fully determined. One short observational study demonstrated the cardiovascular risk of patients prescribed a TNF inhibitor was similar to that of patients who had switched to tocilizumab.[86] Furthermore, in a prospective phase IV cardiovascular outcome trial (ENTRACTE), the risk of incident MACEs was similar in those prescribed tocilizumab compared with patients given etanercept (HR 1.05; 95% CI, 0.77–1.43).[87]

Gout medications Two landmark studies in assessing the inflammatory hypothesis of CVD have focused on the gout treatments canakinumab and colchicine. In CANTOS, directly reducing inflammation with canakinumab, a monoclonal antibody targeting IL-1β, reduced the incidence of recurrent vascular events in individuals with a previous MI and high-sensitivity (hs) CRP greater than or equal to 2 mg/L (HR 0.85; 95% CI, 0.74–0.98; $P = 0.021$), independent of lipid-lowering capacity.[47] Although the benefit-to-risk ratio and cost effectiveness of canakinumab precluded its routine use in clinical practice for secondary prevention of CVD, this study was the first randomized controlled trial to prove the inflammatory hypothesis of CVD.

In the later Colchicine Cardiovascular Outcomes Trial, individuals with a recent MI treated with colchicine demonstrated a 23% RR reduction in the primary composite outcome of death from cardiovascular causes, resuscitated cardiac arrest, MI, stroke, or urgent hospitalization for angina leading to coronary revascularization (HR 0.77; 95% CI, 0.61–0.96; $P = 0.02$) compared with placebo.[88] Overall adverse event rates were similar in colchicine and placebo groups. The primary outcome was driven mainly by a reduction in stroke events and urgent hospitalization for angina leading to revascularization (the latter a softer CVD outcome), with no statistically significant reduction in MI rate or mortality. Therefore, although colchicine may have a potential role in stroke warranting further study, it is not recommended at present as part of routine secondary CVD prevention.[89]

There also has been interest in the potential use of xanthine oxidase inhibitors (XOIs), such as allopurinol, in the treatment of cerebrovascular disease and CVD through reduction of vascular oxidative stress and circulating uric acid levels.[45] Studies in individuals with hyperuricemia and gout have shown mixed effects of

XOIs on CVD outcomes.[90,91] In 2018, the Cardiovascular Safety of Febuxostat and Allopurinol in Patients With Gout and Cardiovascular Comorbidities study compared cardiovascular outcomes between patients with gout and coexisting CVD receiving either febuxostat or allopurinol. Although febuxostat was noninferior to allopurinol with respect to rates of adverse cardiovascular events, all-cause and cardiovascular mortality were higher with febuxostat than with allopurinol, raising potential safety concerns over the use of febuxostat in patients with existing CVD.[92]

SUMMARY

In summary, this article highlights the heightened cardiovascular risk in inflammatory joint disease. This is related to a combination of an increased prevalence of traditional cardiovascular risk factors, disease-specific mechanisms, and certain medications commonly prescribed in RMDs, including some NSAIDs as well as prolonged use of relatively high dose corticosteroids. Although CVD risk appears to be falling in RA, likely related to the availability of better treatments, CVD risk still remains elevated compared with the general population. In SLE, CVD risk remains substantially elevated, particularly in those with longer disease duration, more chronic organ damage, associated lupus nephritis, NSAID/corticosteroid use, and concomitant hypertension/dyslipidemia. Heightened CVD risk in gout likely is related to traditional cardiovascular risk factors, hyperuricemia, and systemic inflammation.

Taken together, it is important to assess total CVD risk in individuals with inflammatory joint disease. At present, in the absence of disease-specific risk prediction algorithms, standard risk calculators, such as SCORE, may be used, with a 1.5 multiplication factor in those with RA suggested by current EULAR guidelines. Treatment should involve addressing traditional CVD risk factors, including hypertension, dyslipidemia, smoking, diabetes, and obesity, with lifestyle interventions and pharmacotherapy as well as dampening inflammation with DMARDs. Medications associated with heightened CVD risk, including certain NSAIDs (notably diclofenac) and some COX-2 inhibitors (namely rofecoxib, now withdrawn from practice), should be avoided. In cases where corticosteroids are needed, the lowest effective dose should be prescribed for the shortest possible duration.

In conclusion, a holistic, multisystem approach is needed in the management of inflammatory joint diseases. This should include targeting underlying joint inflammation not only to minimize disease activity but also to help improve cardiovascular outcomes in conjunction with optimal management of traditional CVD risk factors.

CLINICS CARE POINTS

- RA, gout, and SLE are associated with increased CVD risk compared with the general population.
- This risk is related to a combination of traditional cardiovascular risk factors, including hypertension, smoking, dyslipidemia, diabetes, and obesity, as well as disease-specific factors, including chronic inflammation.
- Common medications, including some nonselective NSAIDs and the COX-2 inhibitor rofecoxib, as well as prolonged courses of relatively high dose corticosteroids, also can contribute to heightened CVD risk in RMDs.

- CVD risk should be assessed using relevant national or international risk assessment tools, for example, SCORE and Framingham score. Some of these general population tools may need to be adapted in RMDs with a multiplication factor.
- Cardiovascular risk management includes pharmacologic and nonpharmacologic management of traditional risk factors as well as tight control of disease activity with disease modifying anti-rheumatic drugs.
- Lifestyle interventions should be encouraged, including healthy eating, regular exercise, and smoking cessation.
- Antihypertensive and lipid-lowering therapies should be prescribed according to national guidelines and risk assessment tools.
- NSAIDs should be used with caution. When required, naproxen appears to have the safest CVD risk profile. Corticosteroids should be prescribed at the lowest effective dose for the shortest possible duration.

ACKNOWLEDGMENT

LDF is a clinical lecturer at the University of Glasgow funded by the Scottish Clinical Research Excellence Development Scheme (SCREDS), NHS Education for Scotland.

REFERENCES

1. Avina-Zubieta JA, Thomas J, Sadatsafavi M, et al. Risk of incident cardiovascular events in patients with rheumatoid arthritis: a meta-analysis of observational studies. Ann Rheum Dis 2012;71(9):1524–9.
2. Hippisley-Cox J, Coupland C, Brindle P. Development and validation of QRISK3 risk prediction algorithms to estimate future risk of cardiovascular disease: prospective cohort study. BMJ 2017;357:j2099.
3. Schieir O, Tosevski C, Glazier RH, et al. Incident myocardial infarction associated with major types of arthritis in the general population: a systematic review and meta-analysis. Ann Rheum Dis 2017;76(8):1396–404.
4. Crowson CS, Rollefstad S, Ikdahl E, et al. Impact of risk factors associated with cardiovascular outcomes in patients with rheumatoid arthritis. Ann Rheum Dis 2018;77(1):48–54.
5. Ogdie A, Yu Y, Haynes K, et al. Risk of major cardiovascular events in patients with psoriatic arthritis, psoriasis and rheumatoid arthritis: a population-based cohort study. Ann Rheum Dis 2014;74(2):326–32.
6. Baghdadi LR, Woodman RJ, Shanahan EM, et al. The impact of traditional cardiovascular risk factors on cardiovascular outcomes in patients with rheumatoid arthritis: A systematic review and meta-analysis. PLoS One 2015;10(2):e0117952.
7. Robertson J, Peters MJ, McInnes IB, et al. Changes in lipid levels with inflammation and therapy in RA: a maturing paradigm. Nat Rev Rheumatol 2013;9(9):513–23.
8. Robertson J, Porter D, Sattar N, et al. Interleukin-6 blockade raises LDL via reduced catabolism rather than via increased synthesis: a cytokine-specific mechanism for cholesterol changes in rheumatoid arthritis. Ann Rheum Dis 2017;76(11):1949–52.
9. van Sijl AM, Peters MJL, Knol DL, et al. The effect of TNF-alpha blocking therapy on lipid levels in rheumatoid arthritis: a meta-analysis. Semin Arthritis Rheum 2011;41(3):393–400.

10. McInnes IB, Thompson L, Giles JT, et al. Effect of interleukin-6 receptor blockade on surrogates of vascular risk in rheumatoid arthritis: MEASURE, a randomised, placebo-controlled study. Ann Rheum Dis 2015;74(4):694–702.

11. McInnes IB, Kim H-Y, Lee S-H, et al. Open-label tofacitinib and double-blind atorvastatin in rheumatoid arthritis patients: a randomised study. Ann Rheum Dis 2014;73(1):124–31.

12. Taylor PC, Kremer JM, Emery P, et al. Lipid profile and effect of statin treatment in pooled phase II and phase III baricitinib studies. Ann Rheum Dis 2018;77(7): 988–95.

13. Charles-Schoeman C, Fleischmann R, Davignon J, et al. Potential mechanisms leading to the abnormal lipid profile in patients with rheumatoid arthritis versus healthy volunteers and reversal by tofacitinib. Arthritis Rheumatol 2015;67(3): 616–25.

14. The Global BMI Mortality Collaboration. Body-mass index and all-cause mortality: individual-participant-data meta-analysis of 239 prospective studies in four continents. Lancet 2016;388(10046):776–86.

15. Wolfe F, Michaud K. Effect of body mass index on mortality and clinical status in rheumatoid arthritis. Arthritis Care Res (Hoboken) 2012;64(10):1471–9.

16. Escalante A, Haas RW, del Rincón I. Paradoxical effect of body mass index on survival in rheumatoid arthritis. Arch Intern Med 2005;165(14):1624.

17. Sattar N, McInnes IB. Debunking the obesity–mortality paradox in RA. Nat Rev Rheumatol 2015;11(8):445–6.

18. Baker JF, Billig E, Michaud K, et al. Weight loss, the obesity paradox, and the risk of death in rheumatoid arthritis. Arthritis Rheumatol 2015;67(7):1711–7.

19. Ajeganova S, Andersson MLE, Frostegård J, et al. Disease factors in early rheumatoid arthritis are associated with differential risks for cardiovascular events and mortality depending on age at onset: A 10-year observational cohort study. J Rheumatol 2013;40(12):1958–66.

20. Arts EEA, Fransen J, Broeder AAD, et al. The effect of disease duration and disease activity on the risk of cardiovascular disease in rheumatoid arthritis patients. Ann Rheum Dis 2015;74(6):998–1003.

21. Myasoedova E, Chandran A, Ilhan B, et al. The role of rheumatoid arthritis (RA) flare and cumulative burden of RA severity in the risk of cardiovascular disease. Ann Rheum Dis 2016;75(3):560–5.

22. Zhang J, Chen L, Delzell E, et al. The association between inflammatory markers, serum lipids and the risk of cardiovascular events in patients with rheumatoid arthritis. Ann Rheum Dis 2014;73(7):1301–8.

23. Innala L, Möller B, Ljung L, et al. Cardiovascular events in early RA are a result of inflammatory burden and traditional risk factors: A five year prospective study. Arthritis Res Ther 2011;13(4):R131.

24. Libby P. Role of Inflammation in Atherosclerosis Associated with Rheumatoid Arthritis. Am J Med 2008;121(10):S21–31.

25. Ferguson LD, Siebert S, McInnes IB, et al. Cardiometabolic comorbidities in RA and PsA: lessons learned and future directions. Nat Rev Rheumatol 2019;15(8): 461–74.

26. Maki-Petaja KM, Elkhawad M, Cheriyan J, et al. Anti-tumor necrosis factor- therapy reduces aortic inflammation and stiffness in patients with rheumatoid arthritis. Circulation 2012;126(21):2473–80.

27. Gonzalez-Juanatey C, Llorca J, Testa A, et al. Increased prevalence of severe subclinical atherosclerotic findings in long-term treated rheumatoid arthritis

patients without clinically evident atherosclerotic disease. Medicine (Baltimore) 2003;82(6):407–13.

28. Karpouzas GA, Malpeso J, Choi T-Y, et al. Prevalence, extent and composition of coronary plaque in patients with rheumatoid arthritis without symptoms or prior diagnosis of coronary artery disease. Ann Rheum Dis 2014;73(10):1797–804.

29. Pundziute G, Schuijf JD, Jukema JW, et al. Evaluation of plaque characteristics in acute coronary syndromes: non-invasive assessment with multi-slice computed tomography and invasive evaluation with intravascular ultrasound radiofrequency data analysis. Eur Heart J 2008;29(19):2373–81.

30. Roubille C, Richer V, Starnino T, et al. The effects of tumour necrosis factor inhibitors, methotrexate, non-steroidal anti-inflammatory drugs and corticosteroids on cardiovascular events in rheumatoid arthritis, psoriasis and psoriatic arthritis: a systematic review and meta-analysis. Ann Rheum Dis 2015;74(3):480–9.

31. Gelber AC. Gout and risk for subsequent coronary heart disease. Arch Intern Med 1997;157(13):1436.

32. Janssens HJEM, van de Lisdonk EH, Bor H, et al. Gout, Just a nasty event or a cardiovascular signal? a study from primary care - PubMed. Fam Pract 2003; 20(4):413–6.

33. Abbott RD, Brand FN, Kannel WB, et al. Gout and coronary heart disease: The framingham study. J Clin Epidemiol 1988;41(3):237–42.

34. Choi HK, Curhan G. Independent impact of gout on mortality and risk for coronary heart disease. Circulation 2007;116(8):894–900.

35. Clarson LE, Hider SL, Belcher J, et al. Increased risk of vascular disease associated with gout: A retrospective, matched cohort study in the UK Clinical Practice Research Datalink. Ann Rheum Dis 2015;74(4):642–7.

36. Bhole V, de Vera M, Rahman MM, et al. Epidemiology of gout in women: Fifty-two-year followup of a prospective cohort. Arthritis Rheum 2010;62(4):1069–76.

37. Stöckl D, Döring A, Thorand B, et al. Reproductive factors and serum uric acid levels in females from the general population: the KORA F4 Study. PLoS One 2012;7(3):e32668.

38. Carr MC. The emergence of the metabolic syndrome with menopause. J Clin Endocrinol Metab 2003;88(6):2404–11.

39. Kim SY, Guevara JP, Kim KM, et al. Hyperuricemia and Coronary Heart Disease: A Systematic Review and Meta-Analysis. Arthritis Care Res 2010;62(2):170–80.

40. Kuwabara M, Niwa K, Hisatome I, et al. Asymptomatic hyperuricemia without co-morbidities predicts cardiometabolic diseases five-year Japanese Cohort Study. Hypertension 2017;69(6):1036–44.

41. Khosla UM, Zharikov S, Finch JL, et al. Hyperuricemia induces endothelial dysfunction. Kidney Int 2005;67(5):1739–42.

42. Maruhashi T, Hisatome I, Kihara Y, et al. Hyperuricemia and endothelial function: From molecular background to clinical perspectives. Atherosclerosis 2018;278: 226–31.

43. Ho WJ, Tsai WP, Yu KH, et al. Association between endothelial dysfunction and hyperuricaemia | Rheumatology | Oxford Academic. Rheumatology (Oxford) 2010;49:1929–34.

44. Prasad M, Matteson EL, Herrmann J, et al. Uric acid is associated with inflammation, coronary microvascular dysfunction, and adverse outcomes in postmenopausal women. Hypertension 2017;69(2):236–42.

45. Higgins P, Ferguson LD, Walters MR. Xanthine oxidase inhibition for the treatment of stroke disease: a novel therapeutic approach. Expert Rev Cardiovasc Ther 2011;9(4):399–401.

46. Martinon F, Pétrilli V, Mayor A, et al. Gout-associated uric acid crystals activate the NALP3 inflammasome. Nature 2006;440(7081):237–41.

47. Ridker PM, Everett BM, Thuren T, et al. Antiinflammatory therapy with canakinumab for atherosclerotic disease. N Engl J Med 2017;377(12):1119–31.

48. Manzi S, Meilahn EN, Rairie JE, et al. Age-specific incidence rates of myocardial infarction and angina in women with systemic lupus erythematosus: comparison with the framingham study. Am J Epidemiol 1997;145(5):408–15.

49. Dregan A, Chowienczyk P, Molokhia M. Cardiovascular and type 2 diabetes morbidity and all-cause mortality among diverse chronic inflammatory disorders. Heart 2017;103(23):1867–73.

50. Manzi S, Selzer F, Sutton-Tyrrell K, et al. Prevalence and risk factors of carotid plaque in women with systemic lupus erythematosus. Arthritis Rheum 1999;42(1):51–60.

51. Roman MJ, Shanker B-A, Davis A, et al. Prevalence and correlates of accelerated atherosclerosis in systemic lupus erythematosus. N Engl J Med 2003;349(25):2399–406.

52. Valero-Gonzalez S, Castejon R, Jimenez-Ortiz C, et al. Increased arterial stiffness is independently associated with metabolic syndrome and damage index in systemic lupus erythematosus patients. Scand J Rheumatol 2014;43(1):54–8.

53. Gustafsson JT, Herlitz Lindberg M, Gunnarsson I, et al. Excess atherosclerosis in systemic lupus erythematosus, - A matter of renal involvement: Case control study of 281 SLE patients and 281 individually matched population controls. PLoS One 2017;12(4):e0174572.

54. Svenungsson E, Gustafsson J, Leonard D, et al. A STAT4 risk allele is associated with ischaemic cerebrovascular events and anti-phospholipid antibodies in systemic lupus erythematosus. Ann Rheum Dis 2010;69(5):834–40.

55. Giannelou M, Mavragani CP. Cardiovascular disease in systemic lupus erythematosus: A comprehensive update. J Autoimmun 2017;82:1–12.

56. Frostegård J, Svenungsson E, Wu R, et al. Lipid peroxidation is enhanced in patients with systemic lupus erythematosus and is associated with arterial and renal disease manifestations. Arthritis Rheum 2005;52(1):192–200.

57. Frostegård J. Systemic lupus erythematosus and cardiovascular disease. Lupus 2008;17(5 SPEC. ISS):364–7.

58. Somers EC, Zhao W, Lewis EE, et al. Type I interferons are associated with subclinical markers of cardiovascular disease in a cohort of systemic lupus erythematosus patients. PLoS One 2012;7(5):e37000.

59. Lewandowski LB, Kaplan MJ. Update on cardiovascular disease in lupus. Curr Opin Rheumatol 2016;28(5):468–76.

60. Mayadas TN, Tsokos GC, Tsuboi N. Mechanisms of immune complex-mediated neutrophil recruitment and tissue injury. Circulation 2009;120(20):2012–24.

61. Arts EEA, Popa C, Den Broeder AA, et al. Performance of four current risk algorithms in predicting cardiovascular events in patients with early rheumatoid arthritis. Ann Rheum Dis 2015;74(4):668–74.

62. Crowson CS, Matteson EL, Roger VL, et al. Usefulness of risk scores to estimate the risk of cardiovascular disease in patients with rheumatoid arthritis. Am J Cardiol 2012;110(3):420–4.

63. Agca R, Heslinga SC, Rollefstad S, et al. EULAR recommendations for cardiovascular disease risk management in patients with rheumatoid arthritis and other forms of inflammatory joint disorders: 2015/2016 update. Ann Rheum Dis 2017;76(1):17–28.

64. Stavropoulos-Kalinoglou A, Metsios GS, Van Zanten JJJCSV, et al. Individualised aerobic and resistance exercise training improves cardiorespiratory fitness and reduces cardiovascular risk in patients with rheumatoid arthritis. Ann Rheum Dis 2013;72(11):1819–25.

65. Metsios GS, Stavropoulos-Kalinoglou A, Van Zanten JJCSV, et al. Individualised exercise improves endothelial function in patients with rheumatoid arthritis. Ann Rheum Dis 2014;73(4):748–51.

66. Ettehad D, Emdin CA, Kiran A, et al. Blood pressure lowering for prevention of cardiovascular disease and death: a systematic review and meta-analysis. Lancet 2016;387(10022):957–67.

67. Baigent C, Keech A, Kearney PM, et al. Efficacy and safety of cholesterol-lowering treatment: prospective meta-analysis of data from 90,056 participants in 14 randomised trials of statins. Lancet 2005;366(9493):1267–78.

68. Kitas GD, Nightingale P, Armitage J, et al. A multicenter, randomized, placebo-controlled trial of atorvastatin for the primary prevention of cardiovascular events in patients with rheumatoid arthritis. Arthritis Rheumatol 2019;71(9):1437–49.

69. Fosbøl E, Gislason G, Jacobsen S, et al. Risk of Myocardial Infarction and Death Associated With the Use of Nonsteroidal Anti-Inflammatory Drugs (NSAIDs) Among Healthy Individuals: A Nationwide Cohort Study. Clin Pharmacol Ther 2009;85(2):190–7.

70. Coxib and traditional NSAID Trialists' (CNT) Collaboration, Bhala N, Emberson J, et al. Vascular and upper gastrointestinal effects of non-steroidal anti-inflammatory drugs: meta-analyses of individual participant data from randomised trials. Lancet 2013;382(9894):769–79.

71. Lindhardsen J, Gislason GH, Jacobsen S, et al. Non-steroidal anti-inflammatory drugs and risk of cardiovascular disease in patients with rheumatoid arthritis: a nationwide cohort study. Ann Rheum Dis 2014;73(8):1515–21.

72. Bresalier RS, Sandler RS, Quan H, et al. Cardiovascular events associated with rofecoxib in a colorectal adenoma chemoprevention trial. N Engl J Med 2005; 352(11):1092–102.

73. Nissen SE, Yeomans ND, Solomon DH, et al. Cardiovascular Safety of Celecoxib, Naproxen, or Ibuprofen for Arthritis. N Engl J Med 2016;2519–29.

74. del Rincón I, Battafarano DF, Restrepo JF, et al. Glucocorticoid dose thresholds associated with all-cause and cardiovascular mortality in rheumatoid arthritis. Arthritis Rheumatol 2014;66(2):264–72.

75. Wilson JC, Sarsour K, Gale S, et al. Incidence and risk of glucocorticoid-associated adverse effects in patients with rheumatoid arthritis. Arthritis Care Res (Hoboken) 2019;71(4):498–511.

76. Panoulas VF, Douglas KMJ, Milionis HJ, et al. Prevalence and associations of hypertension and its control in patients with rheumatoid arthritis. Rheumatology 2007;46(9):1477–82.

77. Hartman L, Rasch LA, Klausch T, et al. Harm, benefit and costs associated with low-dose glucocorticoids added to the treatment strategies for rheumatoid arthritis in elderly patients (GLORIA trial): study protocol for a randomised controlled trial. Trials 2018;19(1):67.

78. Choi HK, Hernán MA, Seeger JD, et al. Methotrexate and mortality in patients with rheumatoid arthritis: a prospective study. Lancet 2002;359(9313):1173–7.

79. Micha R, Imamura F, Wyler von Ballmoos M, et al. Systematic review and meta-analysis of methotrexate use and risk of cardiovascular disease. Am J Cardiol 2011;108(9):1362–70.

80. Ridker PM, Everett BM, Pradhan A, et al. Low-dose methotrexate for the prevention of atherosclerotic events. N Engl J Med 2019;380(8):752–62.
81. Ozen G, Pedro S, Holmqvist ME, et al. Risk of diabetes mellitus associated with disease-modifying antirheumatic drugs and statins in rheumatoid arthritis. Ann Rheum Dis 2017;76(5):848–54.
82. Wasko MCM, Hubert HB, Lingala VB, et al. Hydroxychloroquine and risk of diabetes in patients with rheumatoid arthritis. JAMA 2007;298(2):187.
83. Nam JL, Winthrop KL, van Vollenhoven RF, et al. Current evidence for the management of rheumatoid arthritis with biological disease-modifying antirheumatic drugs: a systematic literature review informing the EULAR recommendations for the management of RA. Ann Rheum Dis 2010;69(6):976–86.
84. Dixon WG, Watson KD, Lunt M, et al. Reduction in the incidence of myocardial infarction in patients with rheumatoid arthritis who respond to anti-tumor necrosis factor alpha therapy: results from the British Society for Rheumatology Biologics Register. Arthritis Rheum 2007;56(9):2905–12.
85. Barnabe C, Martin B-J, Ghali WA. Systematic review and meta-analysis: Anti-tumor necrosis factor α therapy and cardiovascular events in rheumatoid arthritis. Arthritis Care Res (Hoboken) 2011;63(4):522–9.
86. Kim SC, Solomon DH, Rogers JR, et al. Cardiovascular safety of tocilizumab versus tumor necrosis factor inhibitors in patients with rheumatoid arthritis: a multi-database cohort study. Arthritis Rheumatol 2017;69(6):1154–64.
87. Giles JT, Sattar N, Gabriel S, et al. Cardiovascular safety of tocilizumab versus etanercept in rheumatoid arthritis: a randomized controlled trial. Arthritis Rheumatol 2020;72(1):31–40.
88. Tardif JC, Kouz S, Waters DD, et al. Efficacy and safety of low-dose colchicine after myocardial infarction. N Engl J Med 2019;381(26):2497–505.
89. Newby LK. Inflammation as a treatment target after acute myocardial infarction. N Engl J Med 2019;381(26):2562–3.
90. Kim SC, Schneeweiss S, Choudhry N, et al. Effects of xanthine oxidase inhibitors on cardiovascular disease in patients with gout: A cohort study. Am J Med 2015; 128(6):653.e7-16.
91. Larsen KS, Pottegård A, Lindegaard HM, et al. Effect of allopurinol on cardiovascular outcomes in hyperuricemic patients: a cohort study. Am J Med 2016;129(3): 299–306.e2.
92. White WB, Saag KG, Becker MA, et al. Cardiovascular safety of febuxostat or allopurinol in patients with gout. N Engl J Med 2018;378(13):1200–10.

Statin-Associated Myalgias and Muscle Injury— Recognizing and Managing Both While Still Lowering the Low-Density Lipoprotein

Andrew L. Mammen, MD, PhD[a,b,c,*]

KEYWORDS

- Statin • Myalgia • Weakness • Myotoxicity • Myopathy • Autoantibody

KEY POINTS

- Patients who have muscle discomfort attributable to statins, but do not have muscle enzyme elevations or demonstrable weakness, are defined as having statin-associated muscle symptoms (SAMS).
- Those with CK elevations attributable to statins that resolve with discontinuation of the medication are defined as having statin-associated myotoxicity (SAMT).
- Statin-exposed individuals with elevated CK levels, proximal muscle weakness, and antihydroxy-methyl-glutaryl coenzyme A reductase autoantibodies are defined as having statin-associated autoimmune myopathy (SAAM).
- Patients with SAMS or SAMT can be managed by changing the statin regimen or using alternative lipid lowering medications such as ezetimibe or PCKS9 inhibitors.
- Those diagnosed with SAAM usually require chronic immunosuppressive therapy, should not be reexposed to statins, and may be treated with PCSK9 inhibitors if lipid-lowering therapies are indicated.

This article originally appeared in the Medical Clinics of North America, Volume 105, Issue 2, March 2021.

Funding: This work was supported by the Intramural Research Program of the National Institute of Arthritis and Musculoskeletal and Skin Diseases of the National Institutes of Health.

[a] Muscle Disease Unit, Laboratory of Muscle Stem Cells and Gene Regulation, National Institute of Arthritis and Musculoskeletal and Skin Diseases, National Institutes of Health, 50 South Drive, Room 1141, Building 50, MSC 8024, Bethesda, MD 20892, USA; [b] Department of Neurology, Johns Hopkins University School of Medicine, Baltimore, MD, USA; [c] Department of Medicine, Johns Hopkins University School of Medicine, Baltimore, MD, USA

* Muscle Disease Unit, Laboratory of Muscle Stem Cells and Gene Regulation, National Institute of Arthritis and Musculoskeletal and Skin Diseases, National Institutes of Health, 50 South Drive, Room 1141, Building 50, MSC 8024, Bethesda, MD 20892.

E-mail address: andrew.mammen@nih.gov

INTRODUCTION

Hyperlipidemia is a major risk factor for developing cardiovascular disease, the most common cause of death for virtually all populations in the United States. Indeed, nearly 30% of adults in the United States have elevated levels of low-density lipoprotein cholesterol (LDL-C), which doubles the risk for heart attack. Statin medications, which lower cholesterol levels by inhibiting hydroxy-methyl-glutaryl coenzyme A reductase (HMGCR), significantly reduce cardiovascular events. Unfortunately, despite their efficacy, only a fraction of those eligible for statin therapy use one of these cholesterol-lowering drugs. For example, one recent study estimated that of those adults at high risk for cardiovascular disease, nearly half are not taking a statin.[1] Thus, underutilization of statins for managing hypercholesterolemia remains a significant public health concern.

Although statins are generally safe and well tolerated, skeletal muscle side effects, which range from mild myalgias to severe rhabdomyolysis, may limit their use in a significant number of patients. In one telling study that included more than 10,000 current and former statin users, muscle side-effects were reported by 25% and 65%, respectively. Furthermore, nearly two-thirds of former users stopped taking statins because of side effects.[2] With the ultimate aim of optimizing compliance with cholesterol-lowering therapy and thereby reducing the risk of cardiovascular disease, this review describes the different types of statin-associated muscle side effects and provide recommendations about how to manage hypercholesterolemia in patients who experience them.

THE SPECTRUM OF STATIN-RELATED MUSCLE SIDE EFFECTS

The term "statin myopathy" has been used to describe a broad range of muscle problems experienced by patients taking statins. However, this term was poorly defined and did not distinguish between patients who had different symptoms, laboratory findings, and histopathological findings on muscle biopsy. In order to capture the heterogeneity of statin-associated muscle complaints, the National Lipid Association Task Force (NLATF) proposed using more precise terminology in 2014.[3] The term "myalgia" was used to describe muscle discomfort in patients without serum creatine kinase (CK) elevations or objective weakness. Those with "myopathy" have muscle weakness (not attributable to muscle pain) with or without CK elevations. Patients with "myositis" have muscle biopsies revealing inflammatory cell infiltrates. The term "myonecrosis" was used to describe a process that includes significant CK elevations that are at least 3-fold higher than untreated baseline levels or the normative upper limit when adjusted for age, sex, and race. And finally, the term "myonecrosis with myoglobinuria" defines the most severe patients, who have CK elevations along with an increased serum creatine greater than or equal to 0.5 mg/dL and, in some cases, acute renal failure due to precipitation of myoglobin in the kidney tubules (ie, rhabdomyolysis).

Although the NLATF-proposed terminology represents a significant improvement over the vague term "statin myopathy," it does not define mutually exclusive disease categories. For example, a patient with muscle weakness, serum CK elevations, and an inflammatory muscle biopsy could be described as having myopathy, myonecrosis, and myositis. Furthermore, since this terminology scheme was proposed, it has become increasingly clear that statins may trigger an autoimmune myopathy associated with autoantibodies recognizing HMGCR.[4] Given the limitations of the NLATF and other existing classification schemes, the author has found it clinically useful to divide statin-related muscle problems into 3 categories: statin-associated muscle symptoms (SAMS), statin-associated myotoxicity (SAMT), and statin-associated autoimmune myopathy (SAAM) (**Box 1**).

STATIN-ASSOCIATED MUSCLE SYMPTOMS

Patients who experience muscle discomfort, such as myalgias or cramps, without CK elevations or demonstrable muscle weakness can be classified as having SAMS. Although this seems to be the most common type of statin-related muscle problem, estimates of its prevalence have varied widely between studies. For example, in the retrospective and unblinded PRediction of Muscular Risk in Observational Conditions (PRIMO) study, 832 (10.5%) of 7924 hyperlipidemic patients reported muscle pain while on statin therapy.[5] In contrast, a meta-analysis including 26 randomized controlled clinical trials in which muscle symptoms were reported found that these symptoms occurred in 12.7% of statin-treated and 12.4% of placebo-treated subjects ($P = .06$).[6] This study raises 2 points. First, it suggests the possibility that the high rate of muscle symptoms in observational studies may be at least partially due to the fact that patients know and anticipate that muscle pain may be a side effect of statins, an example of the "nocebo effect." Second, it underscores the high prevalence of background nonspecific muscle pain even in patients not on statin therapy. Indeed, this study has been taken by some to suggest that muscle pain alone is rarely, if ever, a consequence of the toxic effect of statins on muscle. However, none of the clinical trials included in the meta-analysis were specifically designed to capture the true prevalence of muscle symptoms in those exposed to statins.

The Effect of Statins on Muscle Performance (STOMP) study was designed, in part, to determine how often muscle pain that occurs in statin-treated patients is directly

---

Box 1
Typical clinical features of the statin-associated muscle conditions

Statin-associated muscle symptoms (SAMS)
  Muscle discomfort present
  Normal manual muscle strength testing
  Normal CK levels
  Resolution with discontinuation of statins
  Recurrence with statin rechallenge
  Lipids managed by changing the statin regimen or using alternative agents

Statin-associated myotoxicity (SAMT)
  Muscle discomfort common
  Muscle weakness possible
  Elevated CK levels present
    Minimal SAMT: CK $\leq$3-fold greater than normal limit
    Mild SAMT: CK >3-fold greater than normal limit
    Moderate SAMT: CK >10-fold greater than normal limit
    Severe SAMT: CK >50-fold greater than normal limit
  Resolution with discontinuation of statins
  Recurrence with statin rechallenge (advisable only in selected patients)
  Lipids managed by changing the statin regimen or using alternative agents

Statin-associated autoimmune myopathy (SAAM)
  Muscle discomfort common
  Muscle weakness common
  Elevated CK levels present (>5-fold greater than normal limit)
  Does not resolve with discontinuation of statins; requires immunosuppression
  Disease flares likely with statin rechallenge (not advised)
  Lipids managed by using a PCSK9 inhibitor

related to the medication. In this study, 420 statin-naïve subjects were treated with either 80 mg of atorvastatin or placebo for 6 months. Among these, 19 statin-treated and 10 placebo-treated subjects reported new muscle pain or cramping that lasted more than 2 weeks, resolved within 2 weeks of treatment cessation, and returned within 4 weeks of treatment reinitiation ($P = .05$).[7] Taken together with data from 2 other double-blind, placebo-controlled studies in which subjects with a history of statin intolerance were treated with statin or placebo, washed out, and then treated with the alternative therapy,[8,9] the STOMP trial suggests that in as many as half of statin-treated patients with muscle discomfort, this symptom is not due to the statin.

Given that there is no definitive diagnostic test to establish whether muscle discomfort can be directly attributed to statin use, physicians must rely on clinical features to determine how likely it is that a patient has SAMS. The location and pattern of muscle symptoms may be informative in that symmetric and proximal symptoms are more likely due to statins than asymmetric and/or distal muscle symptoms. In the authors' experience, SAMS is more often characterized by persistent myalgias than intermittent cramping.[10] In addition, most relevant studies (eg, STOMP) have shown that muscle symptoms tend to occur earlier in patients with verified SAMS than in those with nonspecific muscle symptoms.[7,8] Furthermore, once statins are discontinued, patients with SAMS usually experience a marked improvement in their symptoms within weeks; when symptoms persist longer than 8 weeks, alternative diagnoses should definitely be sought. Finally, once statins have been discontinued and muscle symptoms have resolved, statin rechallenge is likely to provoke muscle symptoms in a relatively short time, most often within 4 weeks. These statin rechallenges, although usually unblinded, are critical for establishing the likelihood that a patient has SAMS.

It is worth noting that statin exposure can cause mild CK elevations, usually within the normal range, even in patients who do not experience muscle symptoms. For example, in the STOMP study, statin-treated patients experienced a 20 IU/L increase in CK over baseline compared with those treated with placebo.[7] And although studies have shown that modest statin-related CK increases may occur more often in those who develop SAMS,[11,12] observing a mild CK increase while on statins may not be specific enough to have diagnostic utility in individual patients.

Based on these clinical observations, a tool known as the Statin-Associated Muscle Symptoms Clinical Index (SAMS-CI; **Fig. 1**) was developed[13] to help clinicians determine the probability of SAMS in statin-treated patients who develop muscle symptoms. Although the SAMS-CI still needs to be validated in large-scale clinical trials, preliminary studies suggest that less than 10% of patients with a score of 4 or less (out of 11 possible points) have SAMS. However, because only half of those with confirmed SAMS had scores of 6 or more, the SAMS-CI seems most useful for identifying those patients least likely to have true SAMS.[10]

Although circumstances may vary, diagnosis of suspected SAMS should usually begin by documenting the location, pattern, and timing of muscle symptoms as detailed on the SAMS-CI. Next, statins should be stopped and the timing of muscle symptom improvement should be documented; failure to improve after 4 to 8 weeks strongly suggests the patient does not have SAMS and alternative causes for the patient's symptoms should be sought. During the statin wash out period, factors that may contribute to the risk of statin intolerance should be eliminated if possible. This includes testing for and treating hypothyroidism and vitamin D deficiency. Assuming that the muscle symptoms do resolve and that the patient meets the American College of Cardiology and the American Heart Association guidelines for initiating treatment with a statin, rechallenging the patient with a statin regimen is an essential component

Statin-Associated Muscle Symptom Clinical Index (SAMS-CI)

Instructions:

- Use with patients who have had muscle symptoms that were new or increased after starting a statin regimen.
- A statin regimen includes any statin at any dose or frequency, including a statin the patient has used previously, at the same or a different dose.
- Muscle symptoms may include aches, cramps, heaviness, discomfort, weakness, or stiffness.
- Interpret overall score in light of other possible causes of the muscle symptoms, such as:

  Recent physical exertion   Hypothyroidism   Concurrent illness
  Changes in exercise patterns   Drug interaction with statin   Underlying muscle disease
- See reverse for Frequently Asked Questions

How many statin regimens has the patient had that involved new or increased muscle symptoms?

One	Two or more
Complete the questions on the left side of this page.	Complete the questions on the right side of this page.

Regarding this statin regimen:

A. Location and pattern of muscle symptoms
(If more than one category applies, record the highest number.)   **Enter score:**

Symmetric, hip flexors or thighs	3
Symmetric, calves	2
Symmetric, proximal upper extremity	2
Asymmetric, intermittent, or not specific to any area	1

B. Timing of muscle symptom onset in relation to starting statin regimen

<4 weeks	3
4–12 weeks	2
>12 weeks	1

C. Timing of muscle symptom improvement after withdrawal of statin
(If patient is still taking statin, stop regimen and monitor symptoms.)

<2 weeks	2
2–4 weeks	1
No improvement after 4 weeks	0

Rechallenge the patient with a statin regimen,
(even if same statin compound or regimen as above)
then complete final question:

D. Timing of recurrence of similar muscle symptoms in relation to starting second regimen

<4 weeks	3
4–12 weeks	1
>12 weeks or similar symptoms did not reoccur	0

Total:
All four scores above must be entered before totaling

Regarding the statin regimen *before* the most recent regimen:

A. Location and pattern of muscle symptoms
(If more than one category applies, record the highest number.)   **Enter score:**

Symmetric, hip flexors or thighs	3
Symmetric, calves	2
Symmetric, proximal upper extremity	2
Asymmetric, intermittent, or not specific to any area	1

B. Timing of muscle symptom onset in relation to starting statin regimen

<4 weeks	3
4–12 weeks	2
>12 weeks	1

C. Timing of muscle symptom improvement after withdrawal of statin

<2 weeks	2
2–4 weeks	1
No improvement after 4 weeks	0

Regarding the *most recent* statin regimen:
(even if same statin compound as above)

D. Timing of recurrence of similar muscle symptoms in relation to starting regimen

<4 weeks	3
4–12 weeks	1
>12 weeks or similar symptoms did not reoccur	0

Total:
All four scores above must be entered before totaling

Interpretation	Total score:	2–6	7–8	9–11
	Likelihood that the patient's muscle symptoms are due to statin use:	Unlikely	Possible	Probable

Fig. 1. The Statin-Associated Muscle Symptom Clinical Index (SAMS-CI). (*From* Rosenson RS, Miller K, Bayliss M, et al. The Statin-Associated Muscle Symptom Clinical Index (SAMS-CI): Revision for Clinical Use, Content Validation, and Inter-rater Reliability. Cardiovasc Drugs Ther 2017;31(2):182; with permission.)

of the diagnostic process. No further workup is required for those who do not experience a return of muscle symptoms with the statin rechallenge. However, in those whose symptoms return, especially if they have SAMS-CI scores of 5 or greater, the statin should be stopped until symptoms resolve and then an alternative statin regimen may be initiated. For example, rosuvastatin, atorvastatin, and pitavastatin have long half-lives and can be given every other day (or even once per week) resulting in a lower weekly dose of statin. Although some patients with SAMS tolerate these lower dose regimens, which may not be inferior to daily dosing to reduce LDL-C and triglyceride levels,[14] it remains to be shown how effectively it reduces the risk of cardiovascular events.

Nonstatin medications should be considered for patients who do not reach their target cholesterol levels after demonstrated intolerance to 2 or 3 different statin regimens. The 2017 Focused Update of the 2016 American College of Cardiology Expert Consensus Decision Pathway provides detailed recommendations for choosing an alternative to statins in different statin-intolerant patient populations.[15] Specific recommendations vary depending on the age of the patient, whether the statin is prescribed for primary or secondary prevention, and the presence of certain comorbidities. In most cases, either ezetimibe or a proprotein convertase subtilisin/kexin type 9 (PCSK9) inhibitor is recommended for statin-intolerant patients who would benefit from a reduction in cholesterol levels. Several studies have shown that these agents are less likely to cause muscle symptoms than statin medications and that patients treated with PCSK9 inhibitors may have even fewer muscle symptoms than those on ezetimibe.[9,16,17]

STATIN-ASSOCIATED MYOTOXICITY

The author defines SAMT as statin-induced CK elevations with or without muscle discomfort and/or weakness. By this definition, SAMT encompasses a broad range of patients, from those with modest asymptomatic CK elevations to those with very high CK elevations, myoglobinuria, weakness, and acute renal failure (ie, rhabdomyolysis). "Minimal" SAMT will be defined when CK elevations are at less than 3-fold higher than untreated baseline levels or the normative upper limit (see[18] for normative values based on sex and race). And in keeping with the NLATF terminology, "mild," "moderate," and "severe" SAMT will be defined by CK levels that are elevated by 3-fold to 10-fold, 10-fold to 50-fold, and greater than 50-fold, respectively.

The risk that an individual will develop SAMT after statin exposure depends on several factors including their age and gender, the type and dose of statin prescribed, the coadministration of other medications, and the presence of genetic susceptibility factors. A 2008 paper published by the Study of the Effectiveness of Additional Reductions in Cholesterol and Homocysteine (SEARCH) Collaborative Group illustrates how multiple factors contribute to the risk of SAMT.[19] In this randomized trial of 12,064 patients with prior myocardial infarction, simvastatin was administered to 6031 patients at a dose of 80 mg each day and to 6033 patients at a dose of 20 mg per day. Although just 8 (0.1%) patients on the lower dose of simvastatin developed SAMT (as defined by CK levels at least 3 times greater than the normal limit or 5 times greater than the baseline), 98 (1.6%) patients on the higher statin dose developed this side effect. Among patients on 80 mg of simvastatin each day, this adverse event was 2.3 times more likely in those older than 65 years and 1.6-times more likely in women than in men. Those with impaired renal function had a 2.4-fold increased risk of SAMT. Furthermore, the concurrent use of amiodarone or calcium channel antagonists resulted in an 8.8-fold and 2.7-fold increased risk of developing SAMT, respectively. Finally, this study demonstrated that the rs3471512C allele of the *SLCO1B1* gene (encoding the solute carrier organic anion transporter family member 1B1 protein) confers significant risk for developing SAMT. Specifically, the risk of developing SAMT during the first year among those taking 80 mg of simvastatin each day was 0.6%, 3%, and 18% for those with 0, 1, and 2 copies of the C allele, respectively. Based on the results of the SEARCH collaborative study, it is now recognized that most patients should be started on a low dose of simvastatin and that amiodarone should be avoided in patients taking simvastatin, especially at higher doses. However, genetic testing is not yet routinely performed to identify those patients at highest risk for SAMT.

In patients with suspected SAMT, the first intervention should be to discontinue the statin and document that the CK level returns to normal or baseline. Of note, although checking a baseline CK level before statin initiation is not currently recommended by most published guidelines, knowing the baseline value for the individual patient can be very helpful in those who develop muscle symptoms. Consequently, some clinicians do favor checking the baseline CK before starting statin therapy. That being said, there is no practical role for subsequent monitoring of CK levels in asymptomatic patients who are on statins.

At the same time that statins are discontinued, alternative diagnoses should also be considered. These include exposure to other potential myotoxins (eg, colchicine), endocrinopathies (eg, hypothyroidism), and idiopathic inflammatory myopathies (eg, inclusion body myositis). In SAMT patients, initial CK level reductions should be expected in the first few weeks after stopping the statin and a return to normal levels should rarely take longer than a month. In the event that the CK continues to increase or does not substantially decrease within this time frame, additional alternative diagnoses should be considered. As these include SAAM (discussed later) and previously unrecognized adult-onset inherited myopathies (eg, acid maltase deficiency), evaluation by a neuromuscular specialist would be recommended.

In those with suspected minimal or mild SAMT, a statin rechallenge could be considered to confirm the diagnosis. Depending on individual circumstances, a statin rechallenge might also be performed in some patients with suspected moderate SAMT. For example, some clinicians would consider a statin rechallenge in a white female patient with a CK of 3000 IU/L who experienced muscle discomfort but no weakness while on a statin. However, the author would not recommend a diagnostic statin rechallenge for those with suspected severe SAMT, especially if the patient suffered from renal dysfunction as part of their initial presentation. Furthermore, any statin rechallenge in a suspected SAMT patient should be done cautiously, using a low-dose statin once per week and slowly increasing the frequency or weekly dose while measuring CK levels at regular intervals. In those with documented SAMT based on CK level increases on rechallenge, or in those for whom statin rechallenge seems too risky, hypercholesterolemia should be managed with alternative agents such as ezetimibe or PCSK9 inhibitors.

STATIN-ASSOCIATED AUTOIMMUNE MYOPATHY

Anti-HMGCR myopathy is a subtype of immune-mediated necrotizing myopathy characterized by the presence of muscle weakness, elevated CK levels, and autoantibodies recognizing HMGCR.[4,20] Although some patients develop anti-HMGCR myopathy without having ever been prescribed a statin, exposure to statins is a significant risk factor for developing anti-HMGCR myopathy, and patients who develop the disease in this context are defined as having SAAM. Of note, SAAM is exceptionally rare and has been estimated to occur in just 2 or 3 of every 100,000 patients treated with these agents.[4] One study suggested that those with preexisting diabetes and/or atorvastatin exposure may be at the greatest risk for this adverse event.[21] Although patients with SAAM typically present with myalgias, symmetric proximal muscle weakness, and CK levels greater than 1000 IU/L,[4] occasional SAAM patients may present with muscle pain and elevated CK levels before muscle weakness becomes apparent. Importantly, SAAM is an autoimmune disease that can be confirmed based on the presence of autoantibodies recognizing HMGCR. Statin-exposed patients with muscle pain, weakness, and/or CK elevations who test negative for anti-HMGCR autoantibodies may have SAMS or SAMT but do not have SAAM.[22,23]

Although anti-HMGCR testing is highly sensitive and specific for SAAM, the test may have a false-positive rate of about 0.5%.[22] To avoid misdiagnosis based on this test, only patients with a relatively high pretest probability of having SAAM should be screened for these autoantibodies. For example, patients without CK elevations should not be tested for anti-HMGCR autoantibodies. Furthermore, patients with minimal or mild CK elevations (<10-fold greater than normal limits) should only be tested for anti-HMGCR autoantibodies if their CK levels do not begin to decline within a few weeks (and eventually normalize) after stopping the statin. In contrast, it may be reasonable to screen for anti-HMGCR autoantibodies on initial presentation in patients who have at least moderate CK elevations (>10-fold greater than normal limits), especially if they are also weak. Of note, patients with elevated CK levels, symmetric proximal muscle weakness, and anti-HMGCR autoantibodies can be diagnosed with SAAM without performing electromyography, muscle imaging, or muscle biopsy.[20]

SAAM is usually a chronic autoimmune disease requiring long-term treatment by an experienced rheumatologist or neurologist. Guidelines recently published by a working group of the European Neuromuscular Center suggest that treatment should begin with corticosteroids along with a second agent such as methotrexate or IVIG.[20] Because IVIG may be effective as monotherapy,[24] this approach may also be considered, especially in patients with diabetes or another contraindication to steroids. Importantly, patients with SAAM should never be rechallenged with statins, which may cause disease flare. Although controlled trials remain to be performed, one case series including 8 subjects with SAAM suggests that PCSK9 inhibitors seem to be safe and effective in this population.[25]

SUMMARY

Although statins are generally safe and well tolerated, some patients experience muscle complaints that can limit their use, leading to an increased risk of cardiovascular events. In this review, diagnostic and management approaches were proposed for 3 major types of statin side effects: SAMS, SAMT, and SAAM. Patients with SAMS, who have muscle discomfort and elevated CK levels, must be diagnosed based on their clinical features and recurrence of symptoms following a statin rechallenge. Making a definite diagnosis of SAMS can be challenging given that many individuals have background nonspecific muscle discomfort; future work to define a biomarker for SAMS would be of great potential clinical utility. Hypercholesterolemia can usually be managed effectively in these patients by using an alternative statin regimen or nonstatin cholesterol-lowering agent. The diagnosis of SAMT is often more straightforward because these patients have high CK levels that recur on statin rechallenge (if deemed safe). These patients also usually tolerate an alternative statin regimen or another type of cholesterol-lowering agent. Finally, patients with SAAM can be diagnosed based on the presence of anti-HMGCR autoantibodies. These patients require immunosuppressive therapy and should not be reexposed to statins. Rather, if indicated, their hypercholesterolemia may be managed with a PCSK9 inhibitor. Fortunately, as shown here, after arriving at the correct diagnosis, it should be possible to effectively manage hypercholesterolemia and reduce the chance of cardiovascular events in patients with each type of statin intolerance.

CLINICS CARE POINTS

- In patients with suspected statin-associated muscle symptoms, a statin rechallenge is required to confirm the diagnosis.
- Statins may cause mild CK elevations, usually within the normal range, even in patients who do not experience muscle symptoms.

In patients with suspected statin-associated myotoxicity, other causes, such as hypothyroidism and inflammatory myopathies, should be excluded.

- Ezetimibe or PCSK9 inhibitors can be used to manage lipid levels in those who cannot tolerate statins.
- Testing for anti-HMGCR autoantibodies should be done in patients who are on statins and have CK levels greater than 1000 IU/L.
- Patients with statin-associated autoimmune myopathy and anti-HMGCR autoantibodies usually require chronic immunosuppression.

DISCLOSURE

None.

REFERENCES

1. Ueda P, Lung TW, Lu Y, et al. Treatment gaps and potential cardiovascular risk reduction from expanded statin use in the US and England. PLoS One 2018;13(3):e0190688.
2. Cohen JD, Brinton EA, Ito MK, et al. Understanding Statin Use in America and Gaps in Patient Education (USAGE): an internet-based survey of 10,138 current and former statin users. J Clin Lipidol 2012;6(3):208–15.
3. Rosenson RS, Baker SK, Jacobson TA, et al, The National Lipid Association's Muscle Safety Expert Panel. An assessment by the Statin Muscle Safety Task Force: 2014 update. J Clin Lipidol 2014;8(3 Suppl):S58–71.
4. Mammen AL. Statin-Associated Autoimmune Myopathy. N Engl J Med 2016; 374(7):664–9.
5. Bruckert E, Hayem G, Dejager S, et al. Mild to moderate muscular symptoms with high-dosage statin therapy in hyperlipidemic patients–the PRIMO study. Cardiovasc Drugs Ther 2005;19(6):403–14.
6. Ganga HV, Slim HB, Thompson PD. A systematic review of statin-induced muscle problems in clinical trials. Am Heart J 2014;168(1):6–15.
7. Parker BA, Capizzi JA, Grimaldi AS, et al. Effect of statins on skeletal muscle function. Circulation 2013;127(1):96–103.
8. Taylor BA, Lorson L, White CM, et al. A randomized trial of coenzyme Q10 in patients with confirmed statin myopathy. Atherosclerosis 2015;238(2):329–35.
9. Nissen SE, Stroes E, Dent-Acosta RE, et al. Efficacy and Tolerability of Evolocumab vs Ezetimibe in Patients With Muscle-Related Statin Intolerance: The GAUSS-3 Randomized Clinical Trial. JAMA 2016;315(15):1580–90.
10. Taylor BA, Sanchez RJ, Jacobson TA, et al. Application of the Statin-Associated Muscle Symptoms-Clinical Index to a Randomized Trial on Statin Myopathy. J Am Coll Cardiol 2017;70(13):1680–1.
11. Ballard KD, Parker BA, Capizzi JA, et al. Increases in creatine kinase with atorvastatin treatment are not associated with decreases in muscular performance. Atherosclerosis 2013;230(1):121–4.

12. Taylor BA, Panza G, Thompson PD. Increased creatine kinase with statin treatment may identify statin-associated muscle symptoms. Int J Cardiol 2016; 209:12–3.
13. Rosenson RS, Miller K, Bayliss M, et al. The Statin-Associated Muscle Symptom Clinical Index (SAMS-CI): Revision for Clinical Use, Content Validation, and Interrater Reliability. Cardiovasc Drugs Ther 2017;31(2):179–86.
14. Juszczyk MA, Seip RL, Thompson PD. Decreasing LDL cholesterol and medication cost with every-other-day statin therapy. Prev Cardiol 2005;8(4):197–9.
15. Lloyd-Jones DM, Morris PB, Ballantyne CM, et al. 2017 Focused Update of the 2016 ACC Expert Consensus Decision Pathway on the Role of Non-Statin Therapies for LDL-Cholesterol Lowering in the Management of Atherosclerotic Cardiovascular Disease Risk: A Report of the American College of Cardiology Task Force on Expert Consensus Decision Pathways. J Am Coll Cardiol 2017;70(14): 1785–822.
16. Moriarty PM, Thompson PD, Cannon CP, et al. Efficacy and safety of alirocumab vs ezetimibe in statin-intolerant patients, with a statin rechallenge arm: The ODYSSEY ALTERNATIVE randomized trial. J Clin Lipidol 2015;9(6):758–69.
17. Stroes E, Colquhoun D, Sullivan D, et al. Anti-PCSK9 antibody effectively lowers cholesterol in patients with statin intolerance: the GAUSS-2 randomized, placebo-controlled phase 3 clinical trial of evolocumab. J Am Coll Cardiol 2014;63(23): 2541–8.
18. George MD, McGill NK, Baker JF. Creatine kinase in the U.S. population: Impact of demographics, comorbidities, and body composition on the normal range. Medicine (Baltimore) 2016;95(33):e4344.
19. Group SC, Link E, Parish S, et al. SLCO1B1 variants and statin-induced myopathy–a genomewide study. N Engl J Med 2008;359(8):789–99.
20. Allenbach Y, Mammen AL, Benveniste O, et al. 224th ENMC International Workshop:: Clinico-sero-pathological classification of immune-mediated necrotizing myopathies Zandvoort, The Netherlands, 14-16 October 2016. Neuromuscul Disord 2018;28(1):87–99.
21. Basharat P, Lahouti AH, Paik JJ, et al. Statin-Induced Anti-HMGCR-Associated Myopathy. J Am Coll Cardiol 2016;68(2):234–5.
22. Mammen AL, Pak K, Williams EK, et al. Rarity of anti-3-hydroxy-3-methylglutaryl-coenzyme A reductase antibodies in statin users, including those with self-limited musculoskeletal side effects. Arthritis Care Res (Hoboken) 2012;64(2):269–72.
23. Floyd JS, Brody JA, Tiniakou E, et al. Absence of anti-HMG-CoA reductase auto-antibodies in severe self-limited statin-related myopathy. Muscle Nerve 2016; 54(1):142–4.
24. Mammen AL, Tiniakou E. Intravenous immune globulin for statin-triggered autoimmune myopathy. N Engl J Med 2015;373(17):1680–2.
25. Tiniakou E, Rivera E, Mammen AL, et al. Use of Proprotein Convertase Subtilisin/ Kexin Type 9 (PCSK9) inhibitors in statin-associated immune mediated necrotizing myopathy: a case-series. Arthritis Rheumatol 2019;71(10):1723–6.

Perioperative Management of Rheumatic Disease and Therapies

Diane Zisa, MD[a], Susan M. Goodman, MD[a,b],*

KEYWORDS

- Rheumatic disease • Perioperative care • Perioperative medication management

KEY POINTS

- Rates of orthopedic surgery use among patients with rheumatic disease remain high despite improvements in diagnosis and treatment.
- Patients with rheumatoid arthritis (RA), systemic lupus erythematous (SLE), and spondyloarthritis (SpA) are complex surgical candidates because of their diseases and their use of immunosuppressant medications and are at higher risk of adverse events after surgery.
- Existing systemic manifestations of the rheumatic diseases must be identified and carefully evaluated by the internist during the preoperative assessment.
- The goal of perioperative management of rheumatic therapies is to balance the risks of infection and delayed wound healing when continued with the potential for disease flare when withheld.
- Optimization of these patients before surgery often requires collaboration among multiple specialists.

INTRODUCTION

Patients with rheumatic disease are undergoing orthopedic procedures in considerable numbers, most often to alleviate pain and restore function after years of accrued joint damage. These are medically complex patients because of the potential organ damage from their diseases and their use of immunosuppressant therapy. Thus, these patients demand careful perioperative management and, often, interdisciplinary collaboration. These therapies constitute a rapidly advancing field, and, as such, the medical providers most often tasked with completing the preoperative consultation may be less experienced in their use. This article presents the relevant considerations to managing this challenging population of patients, particularly those with systemic

This article originally appeared in the Medical Clinics of North America, Volume 105, Issue 2, March 2021.

[a] Hospital for Special Surgery, 535 East 70th Street, New York, NY 10021, USA; [b] Hospital for Special Surgery, Weill Cornell Medicine, 535 East 70th Street, New York, NY 10021, USA

* Corresponding author.

E-mail address: goodmans@hss.edu

lupus erythematous (SLE), rheumatoid arthritis (RA), and spondyloarthritis (SpA), through the perioperative period. Special emphasis is given to the principles surrounding the management of conventional synthetic disease-modifying agents and targeted therapies, including biologics, so as to improve patient outcomes and mitigate postoperative risks.

Scope of the Problem

Major orthopedic surgeries, such as total joint arthroplasties, continue to be highly used procedures among patients with SLE, RA, and SpA despite the substantial advances in diagnosis and treatment.[1–5] More specifically, even with the extensive implementation of the disease-modifying antirheumatic drug (DMARD) methotrexate by 1990, and the arrival of the biologics to the treatment armamentarium by 1998, the rate of large joint arthroplasties for patients with RA has remained high, although surgery seems to have been delayed because patients are now older at the time of arthroplasty.[1,3,6] A recent study using a national database of 13,961 patients with RA in England found that this cohort had approximately double the lifetime risk of knee and hip replacements compared with that of the general population.[2] Similarly high use rates are seen for patients with SLE and SpA, the latter of which includes patients with ankylosing spondylitis (AS), psoriatic arthritis, reactive arthritis, and inflammatory bowel disease–associated arthritis.[3,4]

Although rates of arthroplasty remain high, complications are also higher in these patients than for patients with osteoarthritis (OA), and include infection and hip dislocation, and venous thromboembolism (VTE), acute kidney damage, and cardiac complications in patients with SLE.[7,8] This article discusses the specific risks that are increased in these patients by virtue of their underlying inflammatory diseases and medications. Additionally, it discusses our approach to the preoperative evaluation to address modifiable risk factors and optimize them, when possible, before surgery.

PREOPERATIVE CONSIDERATIONS
Anesthesia

Patients with RA and AS can have cervical spinal involvement that presents challenges for anesthesiologists during intubation for general anesthesia. Cervical spine instability and subluxation in RA is usually seen in association with severe, erosive disease and can be asymptomatic, as demonstrated in a study of 154 patients with RA awaiting orthopedic surgery, in which 44% of them were identified as having cervical spine involvement (subluxation or prior surgical fusion) by radiographs.[9] About one-third of patients with cervical spine subluxations did not report associated symptoms.[9] Although gait and balance may be affected in patients with an unstable spine with spinal cord compression, patients with advanced arthritis of the hip or knee may not report this, but signs of myelopathy, such as hyperreflexia, a positive Babinski reflex, or loss of fine motor function in the hands may point to the diagnosis and is easily checked before surgery. Thus, consideration of preoperative screening cervical spine radiographs (with lateral flexion and extension views) should be given to patients with severe, erosive, highly active, and/or long-standing disease before undergoing anesthesia, because manipulation of an unstable cervical spine can result in spinal cord injury or death.[9,10]

Moreover, patients with severe RA can have involvement of the upper airway, particularly arthritis of the cricoarytenoid joints and temporomandibular joints. Hoarseness in the patient with RA is a clue to involvement of the cricoarytenoid joints. If present, it necessitates preoperative consultation with anesthesiologists for a safe and informed plan of care, because trauma during intubation can lead to severe edema and airway obstruction.[11]

Conversely, patients with AS may suffer from cervical spinal fusion and severe osteoporosis, which increases the risk of fracture during endotracheal intubation. These patients can additionally develop restricted chest wall expansion caused by fusion of the costovertebral joints and thoracic spine, to which they adapt by becoming diaphragmatic breathers.[12] Attention to bowel function postoperatively is important in these patients, because a distended abdomen can prevent the diaphragmatic excursion needed for ventilation.[12]

Cardiopulmonary Disease

Inflammation is now recognized as a contributor to the development of atherosclerotic cardiovascular disease in all populations. Unsurprisingly, patients with SLE, RA, and SpA are at higher risk of cardiovascular disease compared with age- and sex-matched control subjects.[13–16]

Total joint arthroplasties are major surgical procedures with potential cardiopulmonary complications, and patients with underlying cardiovascular disease are at increased risk for poor outcomes. The rate of postoperative myocardial infarction in 7600 inpatient orthopedic operations was reported to be 0.6%, but this rate increased to 6.4% in patients with known or risk factors for ischemic heart disease.[17]

RA was not independently associated with an increase in perioperative cardiac events or death when compared with patients with diabetes mellitus or control subjects in a study of noncardiac surgeries using the Nationwide Inpatient Sample of more than 7 million cases or when compared with patients with OA using a Veterans Affairs database.[18,19] However, a study of Taiwan's National Health Insurance Research database found that patients with SLE undergoing surgery (of which approximately 30% were orthopedic surgeries) had higher 30-day postoperative mortality, and that inpatient care, a likely proxy for active SLE, within 6 months of surgery predicted worse outcomes.[7] However, similar to the RA study, cardiovascular events, particularly acute myocardial infarction, did not differ significantly between the SLE and non-SLE groups.[7] Yet, when evaluating patients with SLE undergoing arthroplasty specifically, patients with SLE had a two-fold to seven-fold increased risk of inhospital mortality postoperatively compared with control subjects.[20] In regard to the spondyloarthropathies, the evidence for increased cardiovascular risk after total joint arthroplasty is mixed, particularly in patients with AS.[21,22] Taken together, although data for increased cardiovascular risk in these patients are clear, the same cannot be said for risk of postoperative cardiac events, particularly in patients with RA.

Arthroplasties are categorized as intermediate risk surgeries, with an associated 1% to 5% incidence of cardiac death and nonfatal myocardial infarction, by the American College of Cardiology/American Heart Association.[23,24] Patients with systemic inflammatory diseases may be unable to perform exercise and activities equivalent to four metabolic equivalent tasks secondary to their accrued joint damage, which limits the ability to accurately assess functional capacity.[24,25] Current risk assessment tools, such as the Revised Cardiac Risk Index, or use of traditional risk factors, such as cholesterol levels, may further underestimate the cardiac risk in these patients.[13,24] It is important to have a high index of suspicion for potential subclinical and asymptomatic cardiac disease in patients with rheumatic disease, particularly in RA and AS, when conducting a preoperative assessment, because patient history and traditional risk assessment algorithms alone may not reflect true cardiac risk. Additional evaluation may include a preoperative stress test, with postoperative troponin screening for subclinical cardiac events.[13]

Finally, pulmonary diseases in patients in rheumatic disease range from the more common entities, such as asthma and chronic obstructive pulmonary disease, to the less frequent, including interstitial lung disease and pulmonary hypertension. The latter, pulmonary hypertension, can be fatal in the perioperative context, particularly after the administration of anesthetic agents.[26] Consultation with cardiology, pulmonology, and anesthesiology preoperatively is imperative to anticipate and mitigate risk in affected patients.[13]

Venous Thromboembolism

Patients with systemic inflammatory diseases have higher risks of VTE, including deep venous thrombosis and pulmonary embolism (PE), compared with the general population, particularly at times of high disease activity.[27–32] A review of a Swedish database of all hospital admissions of patients with an autoimmune disorder found that the risk of PE was high and persists beyond the period immediately after hospitalization; for some conditions, the risk lasts for greater than 10 years.[27] This suggests that hypercoagulability associated with the inflammatory disorder itself is likely responsible aside from traditional VTE risk factors.[27]

As potentially fatal complications of total joint arthroplasties, VTE has received considerable attention by the American Association of Orthopedic Surgeons and the American College of Chest Physicians.[33,34] Perhaps because of this additional diligence, patients with RA have not consistently been found to develop VTE at higher rates after arthroplasties, although they do suffer thrombosis at higher rates for medical hospitalizations.[8,35,36] Rates of deep venous thrombosis and PE after total joint arthroplasty in patients with spondyloarthropathies, particularly AS and psoriatic arthritis, however, are mixed, because studies have demonstrated increased and similar rates compared with OA control subjects.[21,37]

Alternatively, patients with SLE do have elevated postoperative risk of VTE that is highest when SLE is active, as demonstrated in patients with preoperative SLE-related inpatient care within 6 months of surgery.[7,38] Patients with SLE with concomitant antiphospholipid syndrome (APS) are at particular risk for VTE.[39–41] APS is characterized by either venous or arterial thrombosis or pregnancy morbidity in the setting of persistent antiphospholipid antibody positivity.[39–41] Patients with SLE with known antiphospholipid antibody positivity or a positive lupus anticoagulant who do not meet criteria for APS are, like all patients with SLE, treated as high risk for VTE, even if they have no history of thrombosis. Although mild thrombocytopenia may accompany APS, it is not typically severe, and the risk of VTE for these patients is not lessened. The goal in the perioperative setting for patients with APS is to formulate a plan that will decrease the patient's risk of thrombosis by minimizing the time spent off anticoagulation, while simultaneously not increasing bleeding risk.[40] Thus, preoperative communication and cooperation among medical, surgical, and anesthesiology teams is necessary to achieve this delicate balance.

Infection

Overall, infection risk is higher in patients with RA, SpA, and SLE, and susceptibility is multifactorial, including disease activity and severity and the use of immunosuppressive treatments.[25] Infections, including periprosthetic joint infection and surgical site infection (SSI), have been shown to occur more frequently after total joint arthroplasty in patients with RA relative to patients with OA, with risks consistently 50% higher.[8,21,37,42–44] However, analysis of a cohort of validated patients with RA at a major referral center with high RA-specific surgical experience did not find a difference in infection rate between patients with RA and OA at 90 days post total knee arthroplasty, supporting prior work that surgeon experience with patients with RA is potentially a mitigating factor in poor outcomes.[35,45] Nasal colonization with *Staphylococcus aureus* has been recognized as a substantial risk factor for SSI.[46] In a recent study, patients with RA treated with biologic therapies were found to have an increased risk of *S aureus* nasal colonization compared with those with RA not on biologics and patients with OA.[47] Although not considered standard of practice, perioperative decolonization of patients with RA on biologics may be considered to lower the risk of infectious complications.[47] Decolonization protocols include either Bactroban ointment applied to nares for 5 days before surgery, twice a day, or chlorhexidine shower or bath daily for 5 days before surgery and drying with a clean towel. Although there is no definitive proof of an impact of *S aureus* decolonization on SSI, it is reasonable in settings with high risk of infection in immunocompromised patients including orthopedic procedures where arthroplasty hardware is implanted.

Efforts should also be taken to optimally manage psoriatic skin lesions close to the surgical site to minimize infectious complications given the known high rates of bacterial colonization found in psoriatic plaques.[42,48]

Finally, patients with SLE have a significantly higher risk of complications, including infection, after undergoing total hip arthroplasty, but not older patients with SLE undergoing total knee arthroplasty who may have less active disease, when compared with control populations.[38,49–51] When postoperative complications for various surgeries in addition to orthopedic were evaluated in a large cohort of patients with SLE, there were higher rates of septicemia and pneumonia, although not SSI.[7] This suggests that the infection risk may be attributable to the systemic disease.[7,25]

PERIOPERATIVE MANAGEMENT OF RHEUMATIC THERAPIES

In addition to the increased risk of infection in patients with RA and SLE inherent to their altered immune function, these diseases are often managed using immunosuppressive medications, thereby further increasing that risk. These medications are categorized as conventional synthetic DMARD (csDMARD), or as targeted therapies, including biologics and Janus kinase inhibitors, which are agents that selectively target specific mediators involved in the inflammatory process.[25] The use of csDMARDs and biologics, and these classes of drugs in combination, is becoming more prevalent and, surprisingly, use of biologics has not had an impact on need for arthroplasty.[1,52,53] As a result, most patients with RA, SpA, and SLE are using these potent immunosuppressants around the time of surgery.[35,44,52,54] As such, careful attention must be paid to the management of these medications during the preoperative evaluation. The goal of perioperative management of rheumatic therapies is to balance the risks of infection and delayed wound healing when continued with the potential disease flare, and resultant threat to postoperative rehabilitation, when discontinued.

csDMARDs, including hydroxychloroquine, sulfasalazine, leflunomide, and methotrexate, have been studied in the perioperative period and overall seem to be safe.[5,55] An older prospective randomized trial in which patients with RA were randomized to either continue or discontinue methotrexate before elective orthopedic surgery, and then compared with patients with RA who had never been on methotrexate, found that patients who discontinued methotrexate before surgery had higher infection rates and higher flare rates.[56] Studies on the safety of leflunomide perioperatively have been mixed, although current consensus is to continue without interruption.[5,57] Because hydroxychloroquine is not immunosuppressive, it should be continued through the perioperative period.[42]

Although ample data support an increased frequency of infection with the use of biologics in nonsurgical settings, direct evidence on the risks of biologics in the setting of surgery is limited. A meta-analysis that pooled data from 11 articles totaling 3681 patients with recent use of tumor necrosis factor inhibitors and 4310 without recent use found that those with recent tumor necrosis factor inhibitor use had a higher risk of developing SSI at the time of elective orthopedic surgery, but this may reflect the increased severity of RA in those receiving biologics.[55] However, studies using administrative data where careful timing of the interval between biologic infusions and surgery could be determined using billing records have not found a relationship between biologics and postoperative infection, although chronic glucocorticoid use was a significant risk factor for infection.[5,58] Consensus recommendations from the American College of Rheumatology and the American Association of Hip and Knee Surgeons suggest that these therapies should be discontinued before surgery and that the procedure should be scheduled at the end of the dosing cycle for the particular medication, thus minimizing the time off drug before surgery, and restarting as soon as the wound is closed after surgery. Normally, the biologic may be restarted once the wound is healing well without any sign of infection and the sutures have been removed, at a minimum of 14 days after surgery.[5]

For patients with SLE, the severity of the disease manifestations informs the recommendations on continuation or cessation of disease-controlling therapies in the perioperative period. Patients with more severe SLE, characterized by severe cardiopulmonary, renal, hematologic, gastrointestinal, ocular, and/or central nervous system involvement, should continue their medications through the perioperative period given the substantial risk of organ- or life-threatening flare should they be discontinued. However, delaying elective surgery until optimal disease control is achieved should be considered when possible.[5] For those patients with SLE without severe manifestations, medications should be discontinued for 1 week before the scheduled surgical procedure and restarted approximately 3 to 5 days after surgery if there are no signs of infectious complications locally or systemically.[5]

Recognizing the need for a consensus-based approach for the perioperative management of rheumatic therapies, members of the American College of Rheumatology and the American Association of Hip and Knee Surgeons published an evidence-based guideline in 2017 developed for use in the setting of total hip or knee arthroplasty.[5] **Table 1** summarizes the medication recommendations set forth in the guidelines, organized by medication class and discussed briefly previously. It additionally includes recommendations regarding appropriate timing of surgery based on dosing schedule of the biologics. It is important to consider the type of surgery when interpreting these recommendations; in patients undergoing minor procedures, such as arthroscopy, continuing all treatment through the perioperative period may be reasonable. However, this would not apply to procedures in which orthopedic hardware is implanted or procedures with a high risk for infection.

Glucocorticoid Management

Glucocorticoid management in the perioperative setting was also addressed in these guidelines.[5] Glucocorticoids have been conclusively shown to increase the rates of infectious and wound healing complications. In a recent retrospective cohort study using national databases of patients with RA having elective total joint arthroplasty, glucocorticoids were strongly associated with a dose-dependent increase in infectious risk postoperatively, even at modest doses of 5 to 10 mg/d.[58]

As part of the preoperative evaluation, therefore, attention should be focused on optimization of glucocorticoid dosing by tapering the dose before surgery to less

Table 1
Medications included in the American College of Rheumatology/American Association of Hip and Knee Surgeons Guideline for the perioperative management of antirheumatic medication in patients with rheumatic diseases undergoing elective total hip or total knee arthroplasty

DMARDs: Continue These Medications Through Surgery	Dosing Interval	Continue/Withhold
Methotrexate	Weekly	Continue
Sulfasalazine	Once or twice daily	Continue
Hydroxychloroquine	Once or twice daily	Continue
Leflunomide (Arava)	Daily	Continue
Doxycycline	Daily	Continue

BIOLOGICS: Stop These Medications Before Surgery and Schedule Surgery at the End of the Dosing Cycle. Resume Medications at Minimum 14 d After Surgery in the Absence of Wound Healing Problems, Surgical Site Infection, or Systemic Infection.	Dosing Interval	Schedule Surgery (Relative to Last Biologic Dose Administered)
Adalimumab (Humira) 40 mg	Every 2 wk	Week 3
Etanercept (Enbrel) 50 mg or 25 mg	Weekly or twice weekly	Week 2
Golimumab (Simponi) SQ 50mg; IV 2mg/kg	Every 4 wk (SQ) or every 8 wk (IV)	Week 5 Week 9
Infliximab (Remicade) 3-5mg/kg	Every 4, 6, or 8 wk	Week 5, 7, or 9
Abatacept (Orencia) weight-based IV 500-1000mg; SQ 125 mg	Monthly (IV) or weekly (SQ)	Week 5 Week 2
Rituximab (Rituxan) 1000 mg	2 doses 2 wk apart every 4–6 mo	Month 7
Tocilizumab (Actemra) IV 4 mg/kg; SQ 162 mg	Every wk (SQ) or every 4 wk (IV)	Week 2 or Week 5
Anakinra (Kineret) SQ 100 mg	Daily	Day 2
Secukinumab (Cosentyx) 150 mg	Every 4 wk	Week 5
Ustekinumab (Stelara) 45 mg	Every 12 wk	Week 13
Belimumab (Benlysta) IV 10mg/kg	Every 4 wk	Week 5
Tofacitinib (Xeljanz) 5 mg: stop this medication 7 d before surgery	Daily or twice daily	7 d after last dose

SEVERE SLE-SPECIFIC MEDICATIONS: Continue These Medications in the Perioperative Period.	Dosing Interval	Continue/Withhold
Mycophenolate	Twice daily	Continue
Azathioprine	Daily or twice daily	Continue
Cyclosporine	Twice daily	Continue
Tacrolimus	Twice daily (IV and PO)	Continue

NOT-SEVERE SLE: Discontinue These Medications in the Perioperative Period.	Dosing Interval	Continue/Withhold
Mycophenolate	Twice daily	Withhold
Azathioprine	Daily or twice daily	Withhold
Cyclosporine	Twice daily	Withhold
Tacrolimus	Twice daily (IV and PO)	Withhold

Dosing intervals obtained from prescribing information provided online by pharmaceutical companies.

Abbreviations: IV, intravenous; PO, by mouth; SQ, subcutaneous.

From Goodman SM, Springer B, Guyatt G, et al. 2017 American College of Rheumatology/American Association of Hip and Knee Surgeons Guideline for the Perioperative Management of Antirheumatic Medication in Patients with Rheumatic Diseases Undergoing Elective Total Hip or Total Knee Arthroplasty. Arthritis Rheumatol 2017;69(8):1541; with permission.

than 20 mg/d whenever possible.[5] Although pharmacoepidemiologic data support the increase in risk for patients receiving daily glucocorticoid therapy, a decrease in risk with preoperative dose reduction has not been proven.[58] Furthermore, as a challenge to the widely entrenched implementation of "stress-dose" or supraphysiologic dose administration at the time of surgery to avoid adrenal insufficiency with hypotension and shock in chronically glucocorticoid-treated patients, these guidelines suggest that continuation of the patient's usual daily dose of glucocorticoid is generally sufficient in patients undergoing arthroplasty unless the patient began glucocorticoid therapy in childhood. This recommendation is supported by a systematic review on the topic.[5,59,60] As such, usual dosing of glucocorticoids should be continued perioperatively and given on the day of surgery in most arthroplasty surgeries, although prolonged cases or cases under general anesthesia may require additional glucocorticoids. Close monitoring postoperatively for hypotension or alternative signs of adrenocortical insufficiency can prompt administration of additional exogenous glucocorticoid, if necessary. For first case scenarios, where there is concern for drug absorption before starting the surgery, the glucocorticoid dose is administered intravenously in the operating room or holding area.

SUMMARY

Despite advances in treatment, orthopedic surgery for patients with RA, SLE, and SpA remains necessary for a substantial number of patients. These complex patients present challenges in the perioperative period by virtue of their diseases and their immunosuppressant therapies. Multidisciplinary collaboration and thorough evaluations by internists, rheumatologists, surgeons, and anesthesiologists in the preoperative period are therefore necessary for successful outcomes.

CLINICS CARE POINTS

- Cervical spine disease in RA and AS can increase the risk of endotracheal intubation.
- Screening cervical spine flexion/extension radiographs and consultation with an anesthesiologist preoperatively should be considered.
- Patients with SLE are at increased risk for cardiovascular complications after surgery, whereas patients with RA are not, and the risk for those with SpA has not been quantified.

- Cardiac imaging and noninvasive testing may be required to assess preoperative cardiac risk because many patients with RA, SLE, or SpA may not be able to exercise sufficiently to demonstrate their cardiac status.
- Patients with RA do not have higher rates of VTE after arthroplasty.
- Data in patients with SpA are mixed regarding postoperative VTE risk.
- Patients with SLE have a higher risk of postoperative VTE, particularly those with concurrent APS, and thus require careful preoperative planning among specialists.
- Physicians should be aware of the increased risk for infectious complications in patients with SLE, RA, and SpA undergoing total joint arthroplasties.
- csDMARDs can be continued through the perioperative period, whereas targeted therapies including biologics should be discontinued before surgery with surgery planned for the end of the dosing cycle.
- Biologics are restarted when there is evidence of appropriate wound healing with no evidence of infection, typically at approximately 14 days after surgery.
- Minimizing glucocorticoid use before surgery is a critical part of perioperative risk management for patients with rheumatic disease.

DISCLOSURE

S.M. Goodman has research support from Pfizer, Novartis, and Horizon, and has consulted for Pfizer, UCB, and Novartis.

REFERENCES

1. Nikiphorou E, Carpenter L, Morris S, et al. Hand and foot surgery rates in rheumatoid arthritis have declined from 1986 to 2011, but large-joint replacement rates remain unchanged: results from two UK inception cohorts. Arthritis Rheum 2014;66(5):1081–9.
2. Burn E, Edwards CJ, Murray DW, et al. Lifetime risk of knee and hip replacement following a diagnosis of RA: findings from a cohort of 13 961 patients from England [published correction appears in Rheumatology (Oxford). 2019 Nov 1;58(11):2078]. Rheumatology (Oxford) 2019;58(11):1950–4.
3. Mertelsmann-Voss C, Lyman S, Pan TJ, et al. US trends in rates of arthroplasty for inflammatory arthritis including rheumatoid arthritis, juvenile idiopathic arthritis, and spondyloarthritis. Arthritis Rheumatol 2014;66(6):1432–9.
4. Mertelsmann-Voss C, Lyuman S, Pan TJ, et al. Arthroplasty rates are increased among US patients with systemic lupus erythematosus: 1991-2005. J Rheumatol 2014;41(5):867–74.
5. Goodman SM, Spinger B, Guyatt G, et al. 2016 American College of Rheumatology/American Association of Hip and Knee Surgeons Guidelines for the perioperative management of anti-rheumatic medication in patients with rheumatic diseases undergoing elective total hip and knee arthroplasty. Arthritis Rheum 2017;69(8):1538–51.
6. Richter MD, Crowson CS, Matteson EL, et al. Orthopedic surgery among patients with rheumatoid arthritis: a population-based study to identify risk factors, sex differences, and time trends. Arthritis Care Res (Hoboken) 2018;70(10):1546–50.
7. Lin J, Liao C, Lee Y, et al. Adverse outcomes after major surgery in patients with systemic lupus erythematosus: a nationwide population-based study. Ann Rheum Dis 2014;73(9):1646–51.

8. Ravi B, Croxford R, Hollands S, et al. Increased risk of complications following total joint arthroplasty in patients with rheumatoid arthritis. Arthritis Rheumatol 2014;66:254–63.

9. Neva MH, Häkkinen A, Mäkinen H, et al. High prevalence of asymptomatic cervical spine subluxation in patients with rheumatoid arthritis waiting for orthopaedic surgery. Ann Rheum Dis 2006;65(7):884–8.

10. Zhu S, Xu W, Luo Y, et al. Cervical spine involvement risk factors in rheumatoid arthritis: a meta-analysis. Int J Rheum Dis 2017;20(5):541–9.

11. Segebarth PB, Limbird TJ. Perioperative acute upper airway obstruction secondary to severe rheumatoid arthritis. J Arthroplasty 2007;22(6):916–9.

12. Kanathur N, Lee-Chiong T. Pulmonary manifestations of ankylosing spondylitis. Clin Chest Med 2010;31(3):547–54.

13. Goodman SM, Mackenzie CR. Cardiovascular risk in the rheumatic disease patient undergoing orthopedic surgery. Curr Rheumatol Rep 2013;15(354):1–8.

14. Bartels CM, Buhr KA, Goldberg JW, et al. Mortality and cardiovascular burden of systemic lupus erythematosus in a US population-based cohort. J Rheumatol 2014;41(4):680–7.

15. Maradit-Kremers H, Nicola PJ, Crowson CS, et al. Cardiovascular death in rheumatoid arthritis: a population-based study. Arthritis Rheum 2005;52(3):722–32.

16. Wibetoe G, Ikdahl E, Rollefstad S, et al. Cardiovascular disease risk profiles in inflammatory joint disease entities. Arthritis Res Ther 2017;19(1):153.

17. Urban MK, Jules-Elysee K, Loughlin C, et al. The one year incidence of postoperative myocardial infarction in an orthopedic population. HSS J 2008;4(1):76–80.

18. Yazdanyar A, Wasko MC, Kraemer KL, et al. Perioperative all-cause mortality and cardiovascular events in patients with rheumatoid arthritis: comparison with unaffected controls and persons with diabetes mellitus. Arthritis Rheum 2012;64(8):2429–37.

19. Michaud K, Fehringer EV, Garvin K, et al. Rheumatoid arthritis patients are not at increased risk for 30-day cardiovascular events, infections, or mortality after total joint arthroplasty. Arthritis Res Ther 2013;15(6):R195.

20. Domsic RT, Lingala B, Krishnan E. Systemic lupus erythematosus, rheumatoid arthritis, and postarthroplasty mortality: a cross-sectional analysis from the nationwide inpatient sample. J Rheumatol 2010;37(7):1467–72.

21. Schnaser EA, Browne JA, Padgett DE, et al. Perioperative complications in patients with inflammatory arthropathy undergoing total hip arthroplasty. J Arthroplasty 2016;31(10):2286–90.

22. Ward MM. Complications of total hip arthroplasty in patients with ankylosing spondylitis. Arthritis Care Res (Hoboken) 2019;71(8):1101–8.

23. Fleisher LA, Fleischmann KE, Auerbach AD, et al. 2014 ACC/AHA guidelines on perioperative cardiovascular evaluation and care for noncardiac surgery: a report of the American College of Cardiology/American Heart Association Task Force on Practice Guidelines. J Am Coll Cardiol 2014;64(12):e77–137.

24. Fleisher LA, Beckman JA, Brown KA, et al. ACC/AHA 2007 guidelines on perioperative cardiovascular evaluation and care for noncardiac surgery: a report of the American College of Cardiology/American Heart Association Task Force on Practice Guidelines. J Am Coll Cardiol 2007;116(17):e418–500.

25. MacKenzie CR, Goodman SM, Miller AO. The management of surgery and therapy for rheumatic disease. Best Pract Res Clin Rheumatol 2018;32:735–49.

26. Ramakrishna G, Sprung J, Ravi BS, et al. Impact of pulmonary hypertension on the outcomes of noncardiac surgery: predictors of perioperative morbidity and mortality. J Am Coll Cardiol 2005;45(10):1691–9.

27. Zöller B, Li X, Sundquist J, et al. Risk of pulmonary embolism in patients with auto-immune disorders: a nationwide follow-up study from Sweden. Lancet 2012; 379(9812):244–9.

28. Ramagopalan SV, Wotton CJ, Handel AE, et al. Risk of venous thromboembolism in people admitted to hospital with selected immune-mediated diseases: record-linkage study. BMC Med 2011;9:1.

29. Kim SC, Schneeweiss S, Liu J, et al. Risk of venous thromboembolism in patients with rheumatoid arthritis. Arthritis Care Res (Hoboken) 2013;65(10):1600–7.

30. Calvo-Alén J, Toloza SM, Fernández M, et al. Systemic lupus erythematosus in a multiethnic US cohort (LUMINA). XXV. Smoking, older age, disease activity, lupus anticoagulant, and glucocorticoid dose as risk factors for the occurrence of venous thrombosis in lupus patients. Arthritis Rheum 2005;52(7):2060–8.

31. Choi HK, Rho YH, Zhu Y, et al. The risk of pulmonary embolism and deep vein thrombosis in rheumatoid arthritis: a UK population-based outpatient cohort study. Ann Rheum Dis 2013;72(7):1182–7.

32. Chung WS, Lin CL, Chang SN, et al. Systemic lupus erythematosus increases the risks of deep vein thrombosis and pulmonary embolism: a nationwide cohort study. J Thromb Haemost 2014;12(4):452–8.

33. Mont MA, Jacobs JJ, Boggio LN, et al. Preventing venous thromboembolic disease in patients undergoing elective hip and knee arthroplasty. J Am Acad Orthop Surg 2011;19(12):768–76.

34. Falck-Ytter Y, Francis CW, Johanson NA, et al. Prevention of VTE in orthopedic surgery patients: antithrombotic therapy and prevention of thrombosis, 9th ed: American College of Chest Physicians Evidence-Based Clinical Practice Guidelines. Chest 2012;141(2 Suppl):e278S–325S.

35. LoVerde ZJ, Mandl LA, Johnson BK, et al. Rheumatoid arthritis does not increase risk of short-term adverse events after total knee arthroplasty: a retrospective case-control study. J Rheumatol 2015;42(7):1123–30.

36. Matta F, Singala R, Yaekoub AY, et al. Risk of venous thromboembolism with rheumatoid arthritis. Thromb Haemost 2009;101(1):134–8.

37. Cancienne JM, Werner BC, Browne JA. Complications of primary total knee arthroplasty among patients with rheumatoid arthritis, psoriatic arthritis, ankylosing spondylitis, and osteoarthritis. J Am Acad Orthop Surg 2016;24(8):567–74.

38. Roberts JE, Mandl LA, Su EP, et al. Patients with systemic lupus erythematosus have increased risk of short-term adverse events after total hip arthroplasty. J Rheumatol 2016;43(8):1498–502.

39. Miyakis S, Lockshin MD, Atsumi T, et al. International consensus statement on an update of the classification criteria for definite antiphospholipid syndrome (APS). J Thromb Haemost 2006;4:295–306.

40. Saunders KH, Erkan D, Lockshin MD. Perioperative management of antiphospholipid antibody-positive patients. Curr Rheumatol Rep 2014;16(7):426.

41. Pengo V, Ruffatti A, Legnani C, et al. Clinical course of high-risk patients diagnosed with antiphospholipid syndrome. J Thromb Haemost 2010;8(2):237–42.

42. Goodman SM, Figgie M. Lower extremity arthroplasty in patients with inflammatory arthritis: preoperative and perioperative management. J Am Acad Orthop Surg 2013;21(6):355–63.

43. Bongartz T, Halligan CS, Osmon DR, et al. Incidence and risk factors of prosthetic joint infection after total hip or knee replacement in patients with rheumatoid arthritis. Arthritis Rheum 2008;59(12):1713–20.

44. Richardson SS, Kahlenberg CA, Goodman SM, et al. Inflammatory arthritis is a risk factor for multiple complications after total hip arthroplasty: a population-

based comparative study of 68,348 patients. J Arthroplasty 2019;34(6): 1150–4.e2.

45. Ravi B, Croxford R, Austin PC, et al. Increased surgeon experience with rheumatoid arthritis reduces the risk of complications following total joint arthroplasty. Arthritis Rheumatol 2014;66:488–96.

46. Liu Z, Norman G, Iheozor-Ejiofor Z, et al. Nasal decontamination for the prevention of surgical site infection in *Staphylococcus aureus* carriers. Cochrane Database Syst Rev 2017;5(5):CD012462.

47. Goodman SM, Nocon AA, Selemon NA, et al. Increased *Staphylococcus aureus* nasal carriage rates in rheumatoid arthritis patients on biologic therapy. J Arthroplasty 2019;34(5):954–8.

48. Beyer CA, Hanssen AD, Lewallen DG, et al. Primary total knee arthroplasty in patients with psoriasis. J Bone Joint Surg Br 1991;73(2):258–9.

49. Kasturi S, Goodman S. Current perspectives on arthroplasty in systemic lupus erythematosus: rates, outcomes, and adverse events. Curr Rheumatol Rep 2016; 18(9):59.

50. Singh JA, Cleveland JD. Lupus is associated with poorer outcomes after primary total hip arthroplasty [published correction appears in Lupus. 2019 Sep;28(10):1281]. Lupus 2019;28(7):834–42.

51. Singh JA, Cleveland JD. Total knee arthroplasty outcomes in lupus: a study using the US National Inpatient Sample. Rheumatology (Oxford) 2019;58(12):2130–6.

52. Goodman SM, Bass AR. Perioperative medical management for patients with RA, SPA, and SLE undergoing total hip and total knee replacement: a narrative review. BMC Rheumatol 2018;2:2.

53. Hawley S, Ali MS, Cordtz R, et al. Impact of TNF inhibitor therapy on joint replacement rates in rheumatoid arthritis: a matched cohort analysis of BSRBR-RA UK registry data. Rheumatology (Oxford) 2019;58(7):1168–75.

54. Goodman SM, Bykerk VP, DiCarol E, et al. Flares in patients with rheumatoid arthritis after total hip and total knee arthroplasty: rates, characteristics, and risk factors. J Rheumatol 2018;45(5):604–11.

55. Goodman SM, Menon I, Christos PJ, et al. Management of perioperative tumor necrosis factor alpha inhibitors in rheumatoid arthritis patients undergoing arthroplasty: a systematic review and meta-analysis. Rheumatology (Oxford) 2016; 55(3):573–82.

56. Grennan DM, Gray J, Loudon J, et al. Methotrexate and early postoperative complications in patients with rheumatoid arthritis undergoing elective orthopaedic surgery. Ann Rheum Dis 2001;60(3):214–7.

57. Tanaka N, Sakahashi H, Sato E, et al. Examination of the risk of continuous leflunomide treatment on the incidence of infectious complications after joint arthroplasty in patients with rheumatoid arthritis. J Clin Rheumatol 2003;9(2):115–8.

58. George MD, Baker JF, Winthrop K, et al. Risk of biologics and glucocorticoids in patients with rheumatoid arthritis undergoing arthroplasty: a cohort study. Ann Intern Med 2019;170(12):825–36.

59. MacKenzie CR, Goodman SM. Stress dose steroids: myths and perioperative medicine. Curr Rheumatol Rep 2016;18(7):47.

60. Marik PE, Varon J. Requirement of perioperative stress doses of corticosteroids: a systematic review of the literature. Arch Surg 2008;143(12):1222–6.

Fibromyalgia
Recognition and Management in the Primary Care Office

Carmen E. Gota, MD*

KEYWORDS

- Fibromyalgia • Depression • Fatigue • Sleep • Nonpharmacological interventions

KEY POINTS

- Fibromyalgia is a chronic pain disorder resulting from abnormal central sensitization and a chronic stress pattern of response.
- There is no evidence that fibromyalgia is an inflammatory/autoimmune disorder.
- The diagnosis of fibromyalgia is clinically based on a combination of symptoms such as generalized pain, fatigue, nonrestorative sleep, cognitive difficulties, and associated conditions such as irritable bowel syndrome and migraines. Psychological/psychiatric comorbidities are common.
- The evaluation of fibromyalgia should include assessment of mood, sleep, level of exercise, patient maladaptive responses to pain and stressors, and past and present stressors.
- The current available drugs have very limited benefit. The treatment must be individualized and focused on modifying reversible factors: maladaptive responses via psychological interventions, regular exercise, treatment of psychiatric comorbidities, and improvement of sleep.

INTRODUCTION

The medical literature, going back to the nineteenth century, includes numerous writings about what we call today fibromyalgia syndrome (FMS). In 1880, George Miller Beard, an American neurologist described nervous exhaustion or neurasthenia[1] as a medical condition caused by the exhaustion of the central nervous energy reserves, characterized by fatigue, anxiety, headache, depression, shooting pains, local spasms of muscles, and numerous other symptoms that he painstakingly elaborated

This article originally appeared in the Medical Clinics of North America, Volume 105, Issue 2, March 2021.
Case Western Reserve Cleveland Clinic School of Medicine, Cleveland, OH, USA
* Orthopedic and Rheumatologic Institute, Desk A50, 9500 Euclid Avenue, Cleveland, OH 44195.
E-mail address: gotac@ccf.org
Twitter: @gota_md (C.E.G.)

on over the span of 75 pages. In 1904 Sir William Gowers, a British neurologist, coined the name "fibrositis" for a type of spontaneous back pain occurring without evidence for inflammation, aggravated by cold and exertion and associated with sensitivity to mechanical compression, fatigue, and sleep disturbances.[2] Studies of Second World War soldiers reported on "psychogenic rheumatism" and fibrositis as conditions associated with "hysterical features" and "tender localized areas or nodules"[3] intensified and perpetuated by mental influences and persistence despite prolonged bed rest.[4]

Mohammed Yunus used the term "fibromyalgia syndrome" interchangeably with fibrositis to describe the combination of chronic pain, fatigue, stiffness, and poor sleep as a form of nonarticular rheumatism associated with increased tenderness in specific anatomic sites called trigger points.[5]

Fast forward to now, FMS is still defined by its clinical symptoms,[6] largely because the central and peripheral mechanisms of chronic pain are not well understood. Martinez-Lavin described FMS as a stress-related condition resulting from a "failed attempt of our main complex adaptive system to accommodate to a hostile environment."[7] Hans Selye defined stress as a nonspecific response of the body to any demand and coined the term "distress" to describe maladaptive responses to stress leading to somatic and psychological harm.[8] Later Lazarus and Folkman[9] emphasized that the appraisal of a situation, as threatening is important for triggering the stress response with activation of the sympathetic nervous system (fight or flight response) and of the hypothalamic-pituitary-adrenal axis. Several methods of measuring the activation of the sympathetic nervous system such as heart rate variability analysis, tilt table testing, and sympathetic skin response have shown evidence of overactivity in FMS.[10] Both physical (war trauma, surgery, accidents, illnesses, pregnancy and birth, physical abuse) and emotional stressors (sexual and mental abuse, conflict, neglect, divorce) as well as ongoing stressful life events (financial, job, social, family, illness related) have shown long-lasting changes in pain sensitivity, likely via the engagement of the stress response and epigenetic alterations.[11] The exact mechanism of how the activated stress response leads to chronic pain needs further study. Clinical studies show that maladaptive stress responses such as catastrophizing, passive coping strategies, harm avoiding personalities, and depressed and anxious mood perpetuate the stress response, which may contribute to the chronicity of pain.[12] Most recently FMS has been defined as a primary pain syndrome rather than a nociceptive process in the musculoskeletal system[13] largely due to extensive evidence of abnormal brain pain processing[14] and brain connectivity[15] along with malfunction of descending pain inhibitory pathways.[16] Brain studies using functional MRI showed that patients with FMS experience pain and activate brain pain processing areas when exposed to pressure stimuli that are not painful in healthy controls.[14] There is also evidence that peripheral mechanisms may contribute to FMS symptoms such as myalgias and "neuropathic" complaints. Although no structural or inflammatory abnormalities have been observed in peripheral muscles, there is evidence for decreased numbers of small fibers in the skin in patients with FMS[17] and increased levels of glutamate, pyruvate, and lactate in the muscles of patients with FMS that may contribute to the increased pain.[18] This does not rule out the primary nature of FMS pain, as these findings may be the effect of a chronic amplified stress response leading to chronic tissue ischemic changes.

PREVALENCE OF FIBROMYALGIA SYNDROME AND GENDER DISTRIBUTION

The FMS prevalence in the general population is reported between 2% and 10%[19–21] depending on the population studied and the criteria used of diagnosis. Fibromyalgia clinical cohorts often report up to 90% female predominance likely because women are more prone than men to self-refer for care, they have more tender points, and often report more symptoms than men.[22] General population studies using American College of Rheumatology (ACR) diagnostic criteria show ratios of women/men of 6.8 (ACR 1990)[7] to almost equal prevalence (ACR 2016).[10]

DIAGNOSTIC CRITERIA FOR FIBROMYALGIA

The criteria for the diagnosis of FMS have evolved over time.[23–28] The widely used 1990 ACR criteria were focused solely on wide spread pain and the presence of a sufficient number of tender points.[24] Over time the criteria have evolved in several important ways: (1) inclusion of other core FMS symptoms such as fatigue, sleep, and cognitive difficulties; (2) elimination of tender point counts; and (3) allowing exclusively patient completed questionnaires to determine if FMS criteria are met, eliminating the need for a physician input[27] (**Table 1**).

WHEN SHOULD FIBROMYALGIA SYNDROME BE SUSPECTED IN CLINIC?

The diagnosis of FMS is clinical and is often suggested by a "pan positive" review of systems. The core symptoms of FMS are generalized aches and pains often worse with cold and humidity, fatigue, and nonrestorative sleep.[28,29] Other common symptoms are tenderness to touch, stiffness, dryness of mouth and/or eyes, headaches, dizziness, temporomandibular joint complaints, nausea, abdominal pain and bloating, diarrhea often alternating with constipation, frequent urination at night, sensations of subjective swelling, intermittent paresthesias, and environmental sensitivity[5,30] (**Table 2**). Classification criteria for FMS require a minimum of 3 months of symptoms, but most of the patients had symptoms for years, so physicians should be cautious diagnosing FMS in patients with short duration of symptoms, as none of these symptoms are specific for FMS and consider potential "red flags" that may suggest other conditions (**Table 3**). The tenderness to touch defined as sensitivity of soft tissues and muscles to pressure that would not normally cause pain[28] may help differentiate FMS from other inflammatory conditions. About 80% of FMS patients have tender points (areas of increased pain with a standardized pressure of 4 kg/cm^2) on palpation, more often women than men.[22] In 1997 Frederick Wolfe proposed that the tender point count is akin to a "sedimentation rate" for distress and that both fibromyalgia symptoms and tenderness are part of a continuum of distress, rather than discreet diagnostic markers for FMS.[31] The presence of tender points on physical examination is no longer a requirement for diagnosis.[25]

It is not uncommon for patients to resist the passive range of motion and exhibit limited by pain forward lumbar flexion. Occasionally patients also have brisk deep tendon reflexes, cold and purplish discolored extremities, and occasionally a livedoid pattern triggered by cold exposure called cutis marmorata.

COMMON MEDICAL AND PSYCHIATRIC COMORBIDITIES IN FIBROMYALGIA SYNDROME

Patients with FMS are often diagnosed with other conditions presumed to share the common pathophysiology of central sensitization: chronic fatigue, irritable bowel syndrome, pelvic pain syndrome, migraine, temporomandibular disorder, small fiber neuropathy, and interstitial cystitis.[28]

Table 1
Diagnostic/classification criteria for fibromyalgia syndrome

Authors/Citation Name	Criteria	Comments
Wolfe et al,[24] 1990 ACR 1990 FMS Classification Criteria	• Widespread pain • Tenderness at ≥11/18 tender points • Duration of symptoms ≥3 mo	Tender points (24 points, 12 symmetric areas): Upper neck and back • Suboccipital muscles insertion • Low cervical at the level of C5–7 trapezius muscles • Midscapulae Lower back and hips: • Gluteal areas • Greater trochanter areas Anterior chest: • Second rib costochondral junctions • Lateral pectorals at the level of fourth ribs Upper extremities: • Lateral epicondyles lower extremities • Medial fat pad knees
Wolfe et al,[27] 2016 ACR 2016 FMS Criteria	• Generalized pain + pain in ≥4 (out of 5) regions (pain in the jaw, chest, and abdomin are not included) • Duration ≥3 mo • WPI ≥7 and SS ≥5 or WPI 4–6 and SS≥9 • Fibromyalgianess scale = the fibromyalgia severity (FS) scale = WPI + SS; FS scale is a full component of the FMS criteria • A diagnosis of FMS is valid irrespective of other diagnoses	New: • Allows patients with less pain/localized pain extent and more somatic symptoms to be classified as FMS Regions: • Left and right upper region: jaw, shoulder girdle, upper arm, lower arm • Left and right lower region: hip, upper leg, lower leg • Axial region (neck, upper back, lower back, chest, abdomen) WPI measures presence of pain in 19 areas of the body (score 0–19) Symptom Severity (SS) scale assesses 3 key symptoms associated with FMS: fatigue, cognitive problems, and nonrestorative sleep, and other somatic complaints each on a scale from 0-3 (score 0–12) *(continued on next page)*

Table 1 (continued)		
Authors/Citation Name	Criteria	Comments
		The somatic symptom list is simplified to 3 symptoms that have occurred in the past 6 mo: headaches, pain, or cramps in the lower abdomen and depression (each add 1 point if present)

Abbreviation: WPI, Widespread Pain Index.
Adapted from Wolfe F, Smythe HA, Yunus MB, et al. The American College of Rheumatology 1990 Criteria for the Classification of Fibromyalgia. Report of the Multicenter Criteria Committee. Arthritis Rheum 1990;33(2):160-172; and Wolfe F, Clauw DJ, Fitzcharles MA, et al. 2016 Revisions to the 2010/2011 fibromyalgia diagnostic criteria. Semin Arthritis Rheum 2016;46(3):319-329; with permission.

There is a high association between FMS and psychiatric conditions such as major depressive disorder, general anxiety disorder, posttraumatic stress disorder, bipolar disorder, and personality disorders.[28] By using structured clinical psychiatric interviews, criteria for axis I psychiatric disorders were met by at least half, and almost

Table 2 Clinical aspects of fibromyalgia syndrome	
Symptom	Characteristic Features
Pain[32]	Location: • Muscles or joints or both • The back is almost always affected, which helps differentiation from lupus or rheumatoid arthritis that do not affect the lower back Relationship with time of day: • More severe at night, in the morning Relationship with activity: • Worse with prolonged immobility and after exertion Characteristics of pain: • Described in vivid terms: "I feel I have been hit by a truck"; "I feel I have a constant flu"; the pain is "stabbing," "burning," "unbearable"
Stiffness[33]	Duration: • Often longer than 1 h • More pronounced in the morning and after immobility • Does not classically respond to low- to moderate-dose glucocorticoid therapy
Tenderness to touch[28]	• Sensitivity of soft tissues and muscles to pressure that would not normally cause pain[28]
Environmental sensitivity and hypervigilance[28]	• Sensitivity to bright lights and or loud noises and or strong smells • Intolerance to cold and or humidity

Table 3
Conditions to consider in the differential diagnosis of fibromyalgia syndrome

Condition	What Is Common with FMS	What Is Different from FMS
Rheumatoid arthritis and other inflammatory arthritides[32]	• Pain: articular, nocturnal, with rest, better with movement • Stiffness: >1 h • Fatigue • Night sweats ??	• Objective evidence for swollen joints • Abnormal radiographic changes (erosions, chondrocalcinosis) • Lack of low back involvement in rheumatoid arthritis • Elevated markers of inflammation and positive serologies: C-reactive protein, Westergren sedimentation rate, rheumatoid factor, cyclic citrullinated peptide antibodies
Polymyalgia rheumatica/giant cell arteritis[34]	• Pain in neck, upper back, arms, thighs, gluteal area • Stiffness>1 h • scalp sensitivity • Fatigue • Night sweats • Tenderness with palpation over affected areas	• Occurs after age 50 y, often in the 70s • Duration of symptoms of relatively short duration (days, weeks, rarely months) before seeking care • Elevated markers of inflammation • Dramatic response to glucocorticoid therapy • Positive temporal artery biopsy
Inflammatory myositis/dermatomyositis/overlap syndromes/antisynthetase syndrome[35]	• Subjective sense of weakness • Fatigue	• Objective evidence for weakness, proximal and or distal • Lack of myalgias or minimal muscular pain • Elevated creatine kinase (often in the thousands) • Other objective findings: interstitial lung disease, skin rash, periungual changes, occasionally inflammatory arthritis, Raynaud phenomenon
Peripheral neuropathy[36]	• Shooting burning pain • Paresthesias • Numbness • Weakness	• Abnormal neurologic examination • Abnormal EMG
Addison disease[36,37]	• Fatigue • Postural hypotension • Nausea • Vomiting	• Weight loss • Skin hyperpigmentation • Serum cortisol level decreased • Abnormal ACTH stimulation test • Increased eosinophils

(continued on next page)

Table 3 (continued)		
Condition	What Is Common with FMS	What Is Different from FMS
Hypothyroidism[38]	• Fatigue • Cognitive difficulties • Cold intolerance • Constipation • Weight gain	• Hair loss texture change • Goiter • Dry skin • Bradycardia • Decreased deep tendon reflexes • Abnormal thyroid function tests

Abbreviation: ACTH, adrenocorticotropic hormone.

one-third of patients with FMS met diagnosis criteria for axis II.[39] It has been shown that the severity of comorbid depression and the presence of bipolar spectrum symptoms parallel the severity of FMS.[33]

IS LABORATORY TESTING NECESSARY IN FIBROMYALGIA SYNDROME?

Patients with FMS have normal laboratory tests thus blood work is indicated to exclude other conditions that could have similar symptoms and should be limited to hemogram, basic metabolic panel, sedimentation rate, C-reactive protein, and thyroid-stimulating hormone.[40] Routine testing for rheumatoid arthritis or systemic lupus erythematosus is discouraged unless the patient has features to specifically suggest these conditions. In particular, testing for antinuclear antibodies (ANA) can be confusing for the patient because a positive ANA low titer is common in the general population.[41] In particular, ANA tests of low titer less than or equal to 1:160 were found to have a very low (9%) positive predictive value for any connective tissue disease.[42] "At present, ANA positivity occurs so commonly in patients with musculoskeletal complaints and vague symptomatology that a positive results might be neither revealing nor informative: indeed ANA positivity might muddle an otherwise sensible and parsimonious diagnosis work-up."[41]

EVALUATION AND TREATMENT OF THE PATIENT WITH FIBROMYALGIA SYNDROME

Patients diagnosed with FMS are a heterogenous group that require individualized management based on FMS severity and contributing factors.[43]

Education is an essential part of FMS management and should validate the symptoms, reassure, shift focus from symptom management to maintaining function, and emphasize self-pacing and self-management strategies.[44] Patients should be directed to identify their stressors and focus on those who can be eliminated. The University of Michigan Fibro Guide is a free interactive application that uses a cognitive behavioral method to inform and help patients self-manage FMS symptoms.[45] The first step in management should be a graded and stepwise approach prioritizing exercise, mindfulness, and psychological interventions such as cognitive behavioral therapy targeting pain. Finding mental health providers in the community with expertise in cognitive behavioral therapy and interest in FMS can be extremely helpful in managing FMS. Exercise, including aerobic, strengthening, combination of the 2, and mind and body exercises such a Tai chi empower patients to take control and were shown to reduce FMS severity and catastrophizing, improving affect and physical functioning.[46–49]

Table 4
Evaluation and treatment of the patient with fibromyalgia syndrome

Domains	Evaluation	Questionnaires	Approach	Drugs Used in Patients with FMS
Mood	• Prior history of depression, anxiety, other psychiatric conditions • Seeing/seen psychiatry or psychology	• Depression (patient health questionnaire 9) • Anxiety (general anxiety disorder questionnaire) • Bipolar disorder (mood disorders questionnaire)	Mild to moderate: • Counseling • Psychology • Medications: SNRI should be chosen first, but other antidepressants can be tried if SNRI response inadequate or intolerant Severe: • Psychiatric consult	• SNRI • SSRI • Dopamine/norepinephrine reuptake inhibitor • Mood stabilizers
Sleep	• Unrefreshed sleep • Trouble falling and or staying a sleep • Prior history of primary sleep disorders (sleep apnea, narcolepsy, restless legs)		• Sleep hygiene education • Treatment of primary sleep disorders • Sleep medications	• Sleep supplements • Gabapentinoids • Tricyclic/tetracyclic antidepressants • Muscle relaxants
Physical deconditioning	• Moderate exercise at least 30 min 3 times a week		• Education about the role of exercise • Referral to physical therapy	
Stressful life events	• Past stressors: childhood and adulthood physical and sexual abuse, neglect, trauma, illness • Current stressors: financial, family, health, social		• Identify and try to eliminate reversible stressors • Psychological therapy for past trauma • Psychological interventions to change the stress response	
Maladaptive pain responses	• Rumination • Magnification • Helplessness	• Pain catastrophizing questionnaire	• Psychological interventions to address maladaptive pain response	

Patients who do not respond to nonpharmacological interventions may have maladaptive pain responses and/or suffer from sleep disorders and/or active psychiatric conditions (**Table 4**). These patients may require in-depth psychiatric and psychological care, sleep evaluation, and may benefit from added drug therapy.

Many drugs are used to treat FMS, despite poor evidence for efficacy. The Food and Drug Administration (FDA) has approved a gabapentinoid (pregabalin) and 2 serotonin-norepinephrine reuptake inhibitors (SNRI) (duloxetine and milnacipran). Randomized double blind placebo controlled clinical trials in patients with FMS showed that only half of those taking any of these drugs experience a clinically significant (at least 30%) reduction in pain, and the number needed to treat to see a benefit varies between 8 and 14.[50] Similar observations have been made for gabapentin and various other SNRIs and serotonin reuptake inhibitors (SSRIs).[51] There may be subgroups of patients with FMS who benefit more from drug therapy; an SNRI or SSRI drug may be useful in a depressed patient with FMS, whereas a gabapentinoid, a muscle relaxant, or a tricyclic antidepressant at bedtime may be the first choice in those with disturbed sleep. An evaluation for sleep apnea may be helpful in patients with FMS, especially those who are obese. As a general principle if a drug fails to show benefit after 1 to 2 months it should be discontinued. Opioid drugs should not be prescribed for FMS pain.[44]

Patients with severe fibromyalgia such as those who suffer from severe depression, bipolar disorder, or other complex psychiatric conditions and those who catastrophize, take opioids, are refractory to exercise, or seek disability need a much more intensive multidisciplinary care that involves physical therapy, occupational therapy, psychiatry, and psychology.

CLINICS CARE POINTS

- Fibromyalgia is a rule in (not rule out) diagnosis: extensive testing is not required for diagnosis.
- Each patient with fibromyalgia should be evaluated with regard to: stressors, exercise, mood, catastrophizing/maladaptive pain responses, and sleep.
- The treatment of fibromyalgia should be individualized. "One size does not fit all."
- The current FDA approved treatments have limited benefit.
- Medications that are not found effective should be discontinued.
- Nonpharmacologic interventions such as education, exercise, occupational therapy, psychological interventions, and cognitive behavioral therapy should be prioritized.

DISCLOSURE

The author has nothing to disclose.

REFERENCES

1. Beard GM. A practical treatise on Nervous Exhaustion (Neurasthenia). Its symptoms, nature, sequences, treatment. New York: William Wood & Company; 1880.
2. Gowers WR. A Lecture on Lumbago: Its Lessons and Analogues: Delivered at the National Hospital for the Paralysed and Epileptic. Br Med J 1904;1(2246):117–21.

3. Ellman P, Savage OA, Wittkower E, et al. Fibrositis: A Biographical Study of Fifty Civilian and Military Cases, from the Rheumatic Unit, St. Stephen's Hospital (London County Council), and a Military Hospital. Ann Rheum Dis 1942;3(1):56–76.

4. Boland EW, Corr WP. Psychogenic rheumatism. J Am Med Assoc 1943;123(13): 805–9.

5. Yunus M, Masi AT, Calabro JJ, et al. Primary fibromyalgia (fibrositis): clinical study of 50 patients with matched normal controls. Semin Arthritis Rheum 1981;11(1): 151–71.

6. Hauser W, Clauw D, Fitzcharles MA. Fibromyalgia as a chronic primary pain syndrome: issues to discuss. Pain 2019;160(11):2651–2.

7. Martinez-Lavin M. Fibromyalgia: When Distress Becomes (Un)sympathetic Pain. Pain Res Treat 2012;2012:981565.

8. Selye H. What is stress? Metabolism 1956;5(5):525–30.

9. Lazarus R, Folkman S. Stress, appraisal and coping. New York: Springer; 1984.

10. Martinez-Martinez LA, Mora T, Vargas A, et al. Sympathetic nervous system dysfunction in fibromyalgia, chronic fatigue syndrome, irritable bowel syndrome, and interstitial cystitis: a review of case-control studies. J Clin Rheumatol 2014; 20(3):146–50.

11. D'Agnelli S, Arendt-Nielsen L, Gerra MC, et al. Fibromyalgia: Genetics and epigenetics insights may provide the basis for the development of diagnostic biomarkers. Mol Pain 2019;15. 1744806918819944.

12. Nicholas MK, Linton SJ, Watson PJ, et al. Decade of the Flags" Working G. Early identification and management of psychological risk factors ("yellow flags") in patients with low back pain: a reappraisal. Phys Ther 2011;91(5):737–53.

13. Nicholas M, Vlaeyen JWS, Rief W, et al. The IASP classification of chronic pain for ICD-11. Pain 2019;160(1):28–37.

14. Gracely RH, Petzke F, Wolf JM, et al. Functional magnetic resonance imaging evidence of augmented pain processing in fibromyalgia. Arthritis Rheum 2002; 46(5):1333–43.

15. Napadow V, Kim J, Clauw DJ, et al. Decreased intrinsic brain connectivity is associated with reduced clinical pain in fibromyalgia. Arthritis Rheum 2012;64(7): 2398–403.

16. Jensen KB, Kosek E, Petzke F, et al. Evidence of dysfunctional pain inhibition in Fibromyalgia reflected in rACC during provoked pain. Pain 2009;144(1–2): 95–100.

17. Oaklander AL, Herzog ZD, Downs H, et al. Objective evidence that small-fiber polyneuropathy underlies some illnesses currently labeled as fibromyalgia. Pain 2013;154(11):2310–6.

18. Gerdle B, Soderberg K, Salvador Puigvert L, et al. Increased interstitial concentrations of pyruvate and lactate in the trapezius muscle of patients with fibromyalgia: a microdialysis study. J Rehabil Med 2010;42(7):679–87.

19. Wolfe F, Ross K, Anderson J, et al. The prevalence and characteristics of fibromyalgia in the general population. Arthritis Rheum 1995;38:19–28.

20. Wolfe F, Brahler E, Hinz A, et al. Fibromyalgia prevalence, somatic symptom reporting, and the dimensionality of polysymptomatic distress: results from a survey of the general population. Arthritis Care Res (Hoboken) 2013;65(5):777–85.

21. Forseth KO, Gran JT. The prevalence of fibromyalgia among women aged 20-49 years in Arendal, Norway. Scand J Rheumatol 1992;21(2):74–8.

22. Yunus MB. The role of gender in fibromyalgia syndrome. Curr Rheumatol Rep 2001;3(2):128–34.

23. Yunus MB, Masi AT, Aldag JC. Preliminary criteria for primary fibromyalgia syndrome (PFS): multivariate analysis of a consecutive series of PFS, other pain patients, and normal subjects. Clin Exp Rheumatol 1989;7(1):63–9.

24. Wolfe F, Smythe HA, Yunus MB, et al. The American College of Rheumatology 1990 Criteria for the Classification of Fibromyalgia. Report of the Multicenter Criteria Committee. Arthritis Rheum 1990;33(2):160–72.

25. Wolfe F, Clauw DJ, Fitzcharles MA, et al. The American College of Rheumatology preliminary diagnostic criteria for fibromyalgia and measurement of symptom severity. Arthritis Care Res (Hoboken) 2010;62(5):600–10.

26. Wolfe F, Clauw DJ, Fitzcharles MA, et al. Fibromyalgia Criteria and Severity Scales for Clinical and Epidemiological Studies: A Modification of the ACR Preliminary Diagnostic Criteria for Fibromyalgia. J Rheumatol 2011;38(6):1113–22.

27. Wolfe F, Clauw DJ, Fitzcharles MA, et al. 2016 Revisions to the 2010/2011 fibromyalgia diagnostic criteria. Semin Arthritis Rheum 2016;46(3):319–29.

28. Arnold LM, Bennett RM, Crofford LJ, et al. AAPT Diagnostic Criteria for Fibromyalgia. J Pain 2019;20(6):611–28.

29. White KP, Speechley M, Harth M, et al. The London Fibromyalgia Epidemiology Study: the prevalence of fibromyalgia syndrome in London, Ontario. J Rheumatol 1999;26(7):1570–6.

30. Bjorkegren K, Wallander MA, Johansson S, et al. General symptom reporting in female fibromyalgia patients and referents: a population-based case-referent study. BMC Public Health 2009;9:402.

31. Wolfe F. The relation between tender points and fibromyalgia symptom variables: evidence that fibromyalgia is not a discrete disorder in the clinic. Ann Rheum Dis 1997;56(4):268–71.

32. Gota CE. What you can do for your fibromyalgia patient. Cleve Clin J Med 2018; 85(5):367–76.

33. Gota CE, Kaouk S, Wilke WS. The impact of depressive and bipolar symptoms on socioeconomic status, core symptoms, function and severity of fibromyalgia. Int J Rheum Dis 2017;20(3):326–39.

34. Marsman DE, den Broeder N, Boers N, et al. Polymyalgia rheumatica patients with and without elevated baseline acute phase reactants: distinct subgroups of polymyalgia rheumatica? Clin Exp Rheumatol 2020 [Online ahead of print].

35. Clark KEN, Isenberg DA. A review of inflammatory idiopathic myopathy focusing on polymyositis. Eur J Neurol 2018;25(1):13–23.

36. Hughes R. Investigation of peripheral neuropathy. BMJ 2010;341:c6100.

37. Oelkers W. Adrenal insufficiency. N Engl J Med 1996;335(16):1206–12.

38. McDermott MT. In the clinic. Hypothyroidism. Ann Intern Med 2009;151(11): ITC61.

39. Uguz F, Cicek E, Salli A, et al. Axis I and Axis II psychiatric disorders in patients with fibromyalgia. Gen Hosp Psychiatry 2010;32(1):105–7.

40. Arnold LM, Clauw DJ, McCarberg BH, FibroCollaborative. Improving the recognition and diagnosis of fibromyalgia. Mayo Clin Proc 2011;86(5):457–64.

41. Pisetsky DS. Antinuclear antibody testing - misunderstood or misbegotten? Nat Rev Rheumatol 2017;13(8):495–502.

42. Abeles AM, Abeles M. The clinical utility of a positive antinuclear antibody test result. Am J Med 2013;126(4):342–8.

43. Masi AT, Vincent A. A historical and clinical perspective endorsing person-centered management of fibromyalgia syndrome. Curr Rheumatol Rev 2015; 11(2):86–95.

44. Macfarlane GJ, Kronisch C, Dean LE, et al. EULAR revised recommendations for the management of fibromyalgia. Ann Rheum Dis 2017;76(2):318–28.

45. Williams DA, Kuper D, Segar M, et al. Internet-enhanced management of fibromyalgia: a randomized controlled trial. Pain 2010;151(3):694–702.

46. Busch AJ, Webber SC, Brachaniec M, et al. Exercise Therapy for Fibromyalgia. Curr Pain Headache Rep 2011;15(5):358–67.

47. Bidonde J, Busch AJ, Schachter CL, et al. Aerobic exercise training for adults with fibromyalgia. Cochrane Database Syst Rev 2017;(6):CD012700.

48. Pulido-Martos M, Luque-Reca O, Segura-Jiménez V, et al. Physical and psychological paths toward less severe fibromyalgia: A structural equation model. Ann Phys Rehabil Med 2020;63(1):46–52.

49. van Eijk-Hustings Y, Boonen A, Landewe R. A randomized trial of tai chi for fibromyalgia. N Engl J Med 2010;363(23):2266 [author reply: 2266–7].

50. Okifuji A, Gao J, Bokat C, et al. Management of fibromyalgia syndrome in 2016. Pain Manag 2016;6(4):383–400.

51. Welsch P, Uceyler N, Klose P, et al. Serotonin and noradrenaline reuptake inhibitors (SNRIs) for fibromyalgia. Cochrane Database Syst Rev 2018;(2):CD010292.

Management and Cure of Gouty Arthritis

Sarah F. Keller, MD, MA*, Brian F. Mandell, MD, PhD, MACP

KEYWORDS

- Gout • Inflammatory arthritis • Uric acid • Hyperuricemia • Treat-to-target

KEY POINTS

- Gout is a disease of urate deposition; flares are a symptom of the disease.
- In order to stop gout flares, urate deposits must be eliminated with persistent maintenance of low serum urate below the saturation point. A reasonable target is ≤6.0 mg/dL.
- Flare prophylaxis, typically with colchicine or low-dose nonsteroidal anti-inflammatories, should be initiated along with urate-lowering therapy (ULT).
- Do not stop ULT during gout flares or when the patient is admitted to the hospital unless there is a need for absolute liquid and food restriction.
- Treat gout flares until symptoms are completely resolved before tapering or stopping the anti-inflammatory treatment.
- Be aware of comorbidities (such as hypertension, chronic kidney disease, cardiovascular disease, and the metabolic syndrome) and optimize treatment of these conditions.

INTRODUCTION

With a prevalence of 3.9% among all adults, and 9.7% in those older than 80 years, gout is the most common inflammatory arthritis.[1] An analysis of National Health and Nutrition Examination Survey data determined that two-thirds of patients diagnosed with gout do not receive urate-lowering therapy (ULT).[1] As ULT is the only method by which gouty arthritis can be cured, a treat-to-target strategy of lowering serum urate must be widely adopted to optimize care of patients with gout.

GOUT DIAGNOSIS

The gold standard for the diagnosis of gout is the demonstration of monosodium urate (MSU) crystals in synovial fluid or documentation of tophi. Documenting the presence of MSU crystals in the body fluid or tissue is sufficient to diagnose gout. However, because acute gout can occur coincidentally with other types of arthritis, the demonstration of MSU crystals confirms gouty arthritis but does not rule out a concomitant

Department of Rheumatic & Immunologic Diseases, The Cleveland Clinic, 9500 Euclid Avenue A50, Cleveland, OH 44915, USA
* Corresponding author.
E-mail address: kellers@ccf.org

Rheum Dis Clin N Am 48 (2022) 479–492
https://doi.org/10.1016/j.rdc.2022.03.001
0889-857X/22/© 2022 Elsevier Inc. All rights reserved.

septic joint, calcium pyrophosphate arthritis (pseudogout), or another inflammatory arthritis, such as psoriatic arthritis, which can also present acutely in one or a few asymmetric joints. Nonetheless, it is recognized that arthrocentesis with crystal analysis is not always an option.

NONINVASIVE DIAGNOSIS BY CLINICAL ALGORITHM

The diagnosis of gout may be reasonably presumed when joint fluid cannot be obtained based on the patient's specific historical and clinical features or on imaging results. It should be noted (and recorded in the medical record) that without direct documentation of the presence of MSU crystals, the diagnosis is best considered presumptive.

Several clinical algorithms have been developed to assist in gout diagnosis. One diagnostic tool was developed and validated among 328 Dutch patients.[2] Using this algorithm, the probability of gout is graded as low, intermediate, or high based on 7 weighted variables (male sex; previous patient-reported arthritis flare; onset acute and fully developed within 1 day; presence of joint redness; first metatarsal phalangeal joint involvement; hypertension or at least 1 cardiovascular disease [CVD]; and a serum urate level [SUA] >5.88 mg/dL). Additional diagnostic studies (such as joint aspiration or imaging studies) should be used for those patients who fall into the intermediate category or if patients do not follow the expected clinical course. The take-home message supporting the use of such algorithms is that there are characteristic features of gouty arthritis, but they are not 100% specific, which is important to remember when prescribing patients lifelong drug treatment and when assuming that an acutely inflamed joint is not infected.

NONINVASIVE DIAGNOSIS BY IMAGING

The diagnosis of probable gout can be supported by the demonstration of characteristic findings on plain radiographs, musculoskeletal ultrasound (US), computed tomography (CT), and dual-energy computed tomography (DECT). Plain radiographs can be useful in identifying the very late changes of longstanding gout. Gouty erosions tend to be periarticular lesions with sharp, sclerotic margins, which are asymmetric in distribution.[3] These erosions appear as "punched out" of the cortex with pathognomonic "overhanging edges" and "rat bite" appearance.[4] In contrast to the lesions seen in rheumatoid arthritis, mineralization of the periarticular bone and the joint space is typically preserved in gouty arthritis.[3] Tophaceous depositions of MSU crystals are not themselves radiographically opaque, but secondary calcification within the tophus and soft tissue swelling can be evident on a radiograph and support the diagnosis of probable gout.[4] Standard radiography is not a useful diagnostic tool in new cases.[5]

Musculoskeletal US, CT, and DECT have significantly advanced the ability to diagnose probable gout noninvasively, as these modalities have increased sensitivity and reasonable specificity to detect urate deposition. Musculoskeletal US can be used at the point of care in the Rheumatology clinic. Well-established US features of an acute gout flare include occasionally visualizing free MSU crystals within the joint ("snowstorm" appearance) as well as synovial hypertrophy and hypervascularity (as seen by color power Doppler).[5] Deposition of urate can be demonstrated by the "double contour sign," a layer of crystals overlying hyaline articular cartilage.[5] This appearance differs from the intracartilage deposition of calcium pyrophosphate. Gouty erosions and tophi can also be visualized by US. These findings can strongly support the diagnosis of probable gout, but the technique is operator dependent.

CT is an effective modality to image bony deformities, such as erosions and calcified tophi, as these changes can be accurately demonstrated and differentiated from soft tissues based on Hounsfield units.[6] DECT uses 2 different x-ray energies to identify the chemical structure of a given substance based on differences in energy attenuation.[3] In this case, MSU crystals are identified in musculoskeletal structures (eg, joints, tendons, ligaments, muscles) and depicted as a specific color using postprocessing software. As a result, DECT can be used as a method for diagnosing probable gout in the appropriate clinical context. However, although specificity of this modality is high, sensitivity is less than ideal in both acute and tophaceous gout, but it may demonstrate urate deposits in periarticular areas that otherwise might not be detected.[7] Notably, MRI may not reliably distinguish tophus from soft tissue infection.

Although noninvasive approaches can be used when needed, visual crystal documentation remains the gold standard and should be attempted when possible. Synovial fluid analysis with culture should be performed if there is any clinical suspicion for infection.

THERAPEUTIC OPTIONS: TREATMENT OF ACUTE FLARES

Acute flares must be treated while working toward dissolution of urate deposits and cure of gouty arthritis. Nonsteroidal anti-inflammatory drugs (NSAIDs), oral colchicine, glucocorticoids (oral, intramuscular, intraarticular, or intravenous), and interleukin-1 (IL-1) inhibitors can effectively treat gout flares. A critical concept is that flares are a symptom of the underlying disease: the deposition of urate.

According to current society guidelines, NSAIDs, oral colchicine, and glucocorticoids are considered first-line therapies for the treatment of an acute gout attack. IL-1–directed therapy (off-label in the United States) should be considered if there are contraindications to the first-line therapies, or if a patient cannot tolerate or does not respond to the above therapies.[8,9] Choice of agent depends on the patient's preference, response to treatment in the past, and the presence of comorbidities.

Colchicine and NSAIDs are effective, readily available, and reasonably well tolerated. These medications have historically been said to be most effective when initiated within the first 24 to 48 hours of a flare. A potent, generic nonselective COX inhibitor, such as naproxen or indomethacin, is often prescribed at high doses.[10] An open-label randomized trial comparing naproxen to low-dose colchicine in the primary care setting found that there was no difference in initial pain relief between these 2 medications, but naproxen caused fewer side effects.[11] Selective COX-2 inhibitors (such as celecoxib) can be used if there is need to avoid an antiplatelet effect, but higher than the usually prescribed dose may be required.[12] The use of NSAIDs presents a therapeutic challenge, as many gout patients have comorbidities that preclude their safe use.[13] Proton-pump inhibitors should be considered as gastroprotection.[9]

Colchicine can be effective in the treatment of an acute flare, particularly if initiated early during the course of the flare, or if the attack is mild. The trial-based initial dose of colchicine is 1.2 mg followed by 0.6 mg 1 hour later in patients with normal renal function. High-dose oral colchicine (0.6 hourly over 6 hours) is not recommended, as this dosing causes considerably more toxicity than the low dose and provides no greater efficacy.[14,15] As is the case with NSAIDs, caution must be exercised in patients with chronic kidney disease (CKD), as colchicine is largely excreted by the kidney and is not dialyzable. Problematic is that in the clinical trial demonstrating efficacy in relief of pain, resolution of flare was not documented, and most patients required "rescue" pain medication and continued therapy with colchicine.[14]

Chronically used colchicine must be dose-reduced in patients with CKD and particularly those on hemodialysis, if used at all. Importantly, colchicine is metabolized by CYP3A4 and intracellular levels are affected by P-glycoprotein, leading to numerous potentially significant drug-drug interactions.[16]

Glucocorticoids are often used if the patient has not responded to NSAIDs or colchicine, or if there are contraindications to these medications, particularly in the outpatient setting. Several randomized controlled trials (RCTs) have established that glucocorticoids are as effective as NSAIDs for the treatment of acute gout[17,18] and may have fewer short-term side effects.[18] Prednisone or prednisolone can be used at a dose of 20 to 40 mg daily until inflammation has resolved, and then rapidly tapered over the course of 5 to 7 days. If a flare does not resolve with oral glucocorticoids, it is often because the dose was too low, or the therapy was tapered or stopped before complete resolution of flare. Intraarticular glucocorticoids can be considered if only 1 joint is affected and there is no significant concern regarding possible infection.

IL-1–directed therapy is increasingly used, particularly in the inpatient setting. MSU crystals, as well as calcium pyrophosphate dihydrate crystals, activate the NLRP3 inflammasome in mononuclear phagocytes.[15,19,20] This triggers an intracellular cascade of reactions, which results in the release of proinflammatory cytokines, including IL-1β.[15,19,20] IL-1 has proven to be an effective target in treating acute gout. Agents that are directed against IL-1 include canakinumab (a human anti-IL-1β monoclonal antibody approved for treatment of gout in Europe), and the short-acting anakinra (recombinant IL-1 type 1 receptor antagonist). IL-1–directed therapy is well tolerated with very few side effects. Indeed, this class of medication was initially developed to treat sepsis and is thought to be safe for patients in the critical care setting, assuming that any concurrent infection is being treated appropriately.[21]

Several observational and RCTs have demonstrated the efficacy of IL-1 inhibition in treating and preventing gout flares.[22] An RCT investigating the use of anakinra versus intramuscular methylprednisolone in patients with CKD is currently ongoing.[23] Currently, anakinra is the most commonly used treatment by the authors' consult service as therapy for acute gout in hospitalized patients with significant comorbidities (usually some combination of heart failure, diabetes, and renal disease).

TREATMENT OF HYPERURICEMIA: ASYMPTOMATIC HYPERURICEMIA TO ADVANCED GOUT

The overall gout treatment strategy has numerous dimensions: treatment and prophylaxis of acute gout flares, initiation and escalation of ULT, and treatment of associated hyperuricemic-metabolic comorbidities.

In patients with asymptomatic hyperuricemia (>6.8 mg/dL), MSU crystals are potentially silently being deposited in tissues in and around joints (such as tendons and bursae) as well as inside some internal organs. Although there are known risk factors that may predispose a patient with asymptomatic hyperuricemia to develop gout, there is no way to determine with certainty which individual will develop gouty arthritis.[24] Surprisingly, some patients even with profound hyperuricemia (>10 mg/dL) will not develop gout even after 15 years.[25] Treatment of asymptomatic hyperuricemia with ULT is thus not universally recommended, although it can be reasonably considered in certain circumstances.[8] The lifestyle and behavioral changes summarized in later discussion from the American College of Rheumatology (ACR) guidelines are usually recommended for patients with asymptomatic hyperuricemia as well as for all patients with gouty arthritis.[8] These recommendations include weight loss for patients who are overweight (diet, exercise, medications, bariatric surgery),[26] and modifying diet in order to limit intake of purine-rich foods,[27] alcohol and nonalcoholic beers,[28] and high-fructose containing beverages.[29] Last, the patient must be screened for the presence of components of the metabolic syndrome and coronary artery disease.

Flares occur when MSU crystals, presumably originating from tissue urate deposits, trigger an inflammatory response mediated by the NLRP3-inflammasome.[30] Once a gout flare occurs, there is a high likelihood that subsequent flares will recur in the future and will continue to increase in both severity and duration if ULT is not initiated.[24,31] In fact, approximately 90% of patients who experience 1 gout flare will have a subsequent flare at some point in their lifetime.[32] Thus, ULT should be considered. A more conservative therapeutic approach is offered in the ACR gout guidelines: initiate ULT in patients who meet the following criteria (detailed in **Box 1**): clinically or radiologically evident tophi, greater than 2 flares per year, CKD stage $\geq$3, or presence of kidney stones.[8] The authors advocate for a more individualized approach. In certain circumstances, ULT should be strongly considered in patients who may not meet ACR criteria but who would nonetheless benefit from earlier definitive treatment of the underlying disease process to prevent likely progression and put an earlier end to the risk for further gout flares. These patients can include transplant patients, young patients with family history of severe gouty arthritis, or those who experience debilitating, although infrequent flares that negatively impact their quality of life or ability to perform their work.[32] **Fig. 1** details some situations in which ULT should be considered.

Acute flares are followed by periods of time when the disease may appear to be clinically quiet.[24] This "intercritical period" is misleading, as it is during this time that the patient and even the clinician may falsely believe that gout is no longer "active." However, MSU crystals will continue to deposit in tissues, leading to the development of tophi and progression toward destructive arthritis while the threat of triggering a gout attack continues as long as there are urate deposits.[30] ULT is crucial in order to prevent advanced gout, in which patients have chronic joint swelling and pain with potential for joint destruction.[24]

ATTAINING CURE OF GOUTY ARTHRITIS: RATIONALE FOR TREAT-TO-TARGET THERAPY WITH URATE-LOWERING THERAPY

Gouty arthritis is the result of urate deposition from biologic hyperuricemia (>6.8 mg/dL). As total deposited urate cannot be readily measured, serum urate is used as a proxy therapeutic target. In order to cure gout, serum urate must be targeted therapeutically and kept low enough to drive the dissolution of urate deposits by mass

---

Box 1
When to initiate urate-lowering therapy

- Two or more flares per year
- Presence of tophi
- If <2 flares per year, ULT should be considered in an effort to stop future flares in the following cases:
  - Presence of kidney stones
  - CKD stage $\geq$3 (as treatment of flares becomes more difficult)
  - Other conditions making the treatment of acute gout flares unsafe or difficult
  - Significant socioeconomic or medical challenges caused by gout attacks

Data from Pillinger MH, Mandell BF. Therapeutic approaches in the treatment of gout. Semin Arthritis Rheum 2020;50(3):S24-S30.

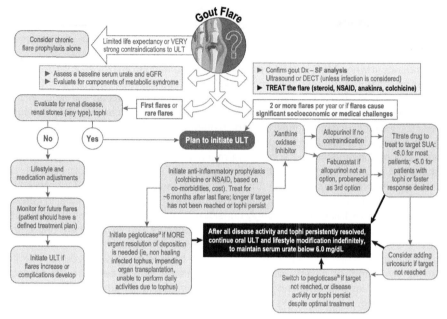

Fig. 1. Management of gout algorithm. DECT, dual energy CT scan; Dx, diagnosis; SF, synovial fluid; SUA, serum urate level; ULT, urate lowering therapy. [a]Do not use other ULT with pegloticase; monitor SUA before each infusion. (*From* Pillinger MH, Mandell BF. Therapeutic approaches in the treatment of gout. Semin Arthritis Rheum 2020;50(3):S26; with permission.)

action effect down a concentration gradient. The lower the serum urate, the more rapid the resorption of deposits.

The saturation point of urate in serum is ~6.8 mg/dL.[24] Any elevation above this solubility concentration will lead to supersaturation and the potential continued precipitation of MSU crystals out of serum and into soft tissue.[24,30] Of note, the upper limit of normal for serum urate as defined by the clinical laboratory is higher than 6.8 mg/dL, meaning that a patient who in fact has biologic hyperuricemia may be mistakenly considered as having "normal" serum urate on population (not biologically) -based laboratory values.[24] For this reason, serum urate should be lowered well below the solubility concentration. A commonly accepted therapeutic target for serum urate is less than 6.0 mg/dL for patients without tophaceous gout, and less than 5.0 mg/dL for patients with clinically or radiographically evident tophi: the concept incorporated into several guidelines is that more extensive deposition represented by palpable tophi warrants more aggressive therapy to promote more rapid dissolution.

There is ample evidence, in the form of retrospective and prospective data, to support ULT in a treat-to-target approach. The optimal range of serum urate concentration to avoid gout flares was determined to be 4.6 to 6.6 mg/dL according to 1 analysis of retrospective data.[33] Another retrospective study demonstrated that reducing serum urate ultimately was associated with a significantly reduced risk of gout flares. Notably, among patients who had average serum urate concentration less than 6 mg/dL, 86% (71 patients) did not have gout flares during the follow-up period of 3 years.[31] A recent large randomized double-blind clinical trial compared allopurinol and febuxostat head to head in the treatment of gout patients and demonstrated that both urate-lowering agents were highly effective when used in a treat-to-target approach. Most patients in both treatment groups did not have flares during the observation period of 49 to 72 weeks following initiation of ULT; only 35% of patients treated with allopurinol had *more than one* flare.[34] Prospective data regarding the benefits of extreme ULT are additionally available from the 2 phase 3 RCTs that investigated efficacy and tolerability of pegloticase (enzyme replacement therapy that metabolizes urate to allantoin). Among patients with elevated serum urate, the use of pegloticase resulted in lower serum urate (primary study endpoint; often to levels $\leq$0.2 mg/dL), as well as reduction in proportion of patients with gout flare and nonstatistically significant reduction in number of flares in biweekly pegloticase group when compared with the placebo group during months 4 to 6 of the study.[35] An analysis of 2 RCTs demonstrated that significantly fewer patients with SUA less than 6 mg/dL experienced gout flares when compared with patients who had serum rate greater than 6.0 mg/dL.[36] There are sufficient direct and indirect data to support the treat-to-target approach.

A critical concept is that when urate lowering is initiated, flares may occur at an increased rate. The benefit of ULT on reducing and ending flares takes time; thus, in the above studies, flare rate was determined months after initiation of therapy.

CONSIDERATIONS IN PATIENTS WITH ASYMPTOMATIC HYPERURICEMIA AND CHRONIC KIDNEY DISEASE

It has long been known that renal function is frequently abnormal in patients with hyperuricemia and gout.[37,38] Elevated serum urate leads to MSU crystal deposition, tophi formation, advanced gouty arthritis, and uric acid kidney stones and is associated with progression of CKD.[37] Several observational studies demonstrated that patients with gout and nongout conditions on ULT had significantly less progression to chronic renal impairment compared with those not on therapy.[39–41] Two large observational studies in Japan have highlighted the association between hyperuricemia and progression of CKD.[42,43] Although these and other studies have demonstrated that lowering serum urate in patients with CKD prevents progression of renal disease, no large RCT has shown that lowering serum urate among those with asymptomatic hyperuricemia prevents development of CKD. Two recent prospective studies in patients with established significant CKD showed no benefit of ULT on slowing progression of CKD.[44]

CONSIDERATIONS IN GOUT PATIENTS WITH CARDIOVASCULAR DISEASE

Gout is associated with an increased risk for presence and death from CVD.[45] However, it has also been demonstrated that chronically elevated serum urate greater than 0.36 mmol/L (6.0 mg/dL) is associated with increased total and cardiovascular mortality among patients with gout.[46] These data raise the question whether reducing gout flares or hyperuricemia with ULT will improve outcome from CVD and emphasize the need to treat aggressively the traditional CVD risk factors in patients with gout.

There is a connection between hyperuricemia and increased cardiovascular risk among patients who are not traditionally considered "high risk" from the perspective of CVD in the general population.[47,48] One large prospective study found that hyperuricemia was an independent risk factor of mortality from total CVD and ischemic stroke in the Taiwanese general population.[48]

AGENT SELECTION AND INITIATION OF URATE-LOWERING THERAPY

The authors' approach to ULT is outlined in **Fig. 1**.[49] There are several agents that can be used in ULT. Once an agent is selected, serum urate should be checked on a regular basis, and ULT should be increased incrementally until the serum urate is at goal (at least <6.0 mg/dL for most patients, <5.0 mg/dL for patients when more aggressive urate lowering is desired). More aggressive therapy is indicated when a more rapid dissolution of urate deposits is desired. If a patient develops a gout flare, the acute attack should be treated, and ULT should NOT be discontinued.

Xanthine oxidase inhibitors are recommended as first-line urate-lowering agents, with a general preference for allopurinol over febuxostat based on cost and historical experience if no contraindication to allopurinol exists.[49] Allopurinol can likely be used safely, even in patients with CKD, as long as it is started at a low dose (50 mg daily) and increased slowly until target serum urate is reached. There should not be any reluctance to increase allopurinol in patients with CKD; dose escalation is seemingly tolerated as long as it is done slowly.[50] The most feared adverse effect is allopurinol hypersensitivity syndrome (AHS), a rare, but potentially fatal cutaneous reaction.[51] This occurs at a rate of a few per 1000 treated patients and is more common in patients with CKD. Although postulated that this is due to a buildup of renally excreted allopurinol or its active metabolite oxypurinol, this has never been convincingly demonstrated. Asians (particular patients of Han Chinese descent) have an increased risk of AHS.[51] African Americans also have an increased risk, and 1 prospective study demonstrated that both Asians and African Americans have a 3-fold increased risk of developing AHS compared with whites and Hispanics.[52] Risk for AHS has been linked to the presence of the HLA-B*5801 allele, and recent ACR guidelines recommend testing for the HLA-B*5801 allele in Asian and African American patients before starting allopurinol.[8] Additional risk factors for AHS include age greater than 60 years, presence of CKD, and starting allopurinol at greater than 100 mg daily.[52,53] There are studies reporting that starting low doses of allopurinol ($\leq$100 mg daily) will permit subsequent escalation to reach the target SUA while preventing the hypersensitivity reaction. Given the rarity of this serious adverse reaction, small studies cannot assure total safety. However, notably, there are no direct studies demonstrating that dose reduction of allopurinol will prevent this reaction and following previously proposed dose reductions of allopurinol in the setting of CKD will not permit therapeutic lowering of the SUA in many patients.

Febuxostat, a nonpurine inhibitor of xanthine oxidase, can be used for ULT if there are contraindications to allopurinol, including a prior allergic reaction to allopurinol.[49,54] As is the case with allopurinol, the lowest dose should be initiated, with incremental dose increases until the target serum urate is reached. Lowering the SUA slowly is less likely to induce flares in gouty arthritis from the rapid dissolution of the deposits. The US Food and Drug Administration issued a black-box alert that febuxostat increases the risk of death when compared with allopurinol and should only be used in gout patients who do not tolerate allopurinol. The authors think that this recommendation was reached based on limited data, including observational studies and an RCT of patients with known significant coronary artery disease, which showed that all-cause mortality and cardiovascular mortality were higher among patients on febuxostat than among patients on allopurinol, whereas overall rates of major cardiovascular events were similar between the 2 groups.[55] There are several significant critiques of the conduct and analysis of this RCT (CARE trial), including a large lost-to-follow-up rate, an imbalance in patients on aspirin between the groups, and the absence of any control group. No good biological explanation is known for this result. A subsequent large prospective noninferiority trial evaluating febuxostat versus allopurinol in the treatment of gout patients demonstrated that the long-term use of febuxostat was not associated with an increased risk of death or cardiovascular events compared with allopurinol.[56] In addition, several other studies completed since the CARES trial have not reproduced the result. Given limited therapeutic options for gout patients who require ULT and the potential for adverse metabolic events owing to untreated hyperuricemia, the authors think that selective use of febuxostat is still warranted if contraindications to allopurinol exist. CKD alone does not mandate therapy with febuxostat, even though it is not primarily eliminated via renal excretion.

If a patient fails to achieve target serum urate on xanthine oxidase inhibitors, a uricosuric agent such as probenecid can be added if the patient has reasonable renal function.[38,49,57] Potent uricosurics are generally avoided in patients with a history of kidney stones. Even if there is no history of renal stones, adequate fluid intake is recommended to prevent nephrolithiasis. Probenecid monotherapy can be used; however, this therapeutic strategy may not be effective if serum urate is markedly elevated or if there is renal insufficiency. Lesinurad has been approved as uricosuric therapy in combination with a xanthine oxidase inhibitor,[57] but is currently not available in the United States. Enzyme (uricase) replacement therapy with pegloticase should be considered in specific situations, as discussed later.

ANTI-INFLAMMATORY PROPHYLAXIS

As can be seen in **Fig. 1**, anti-inflammatory prophylaxis should be initiated before or simultaneously with ULT whenever possible in order to decrease the chance of the drop in SUA precipitating a "mobilization" flare in gouty arthritis.[49] Anti-inflammatory prophylaxis should generally be continued for at least 6 months after the last flare, and typically for longer periods of time if target serum urate is not achieved or if the patient has persistent flares or palpable tophi.[49] Gout flares occur as urate levels change during the titration of ULT, and this can provide impetus for the patient to discontinue ULT unless this phenomenon is well explained in advance.

The choice of prophylactic agent, colchicine or low- to moderate-dose NSAID, is determined based on patient comorbidities and cost.[49] In cases whereby there are contraindications to both NSAIDs and colchicine, low-dose prednisone can be considered, although evidence for this is not available, and anecdotally this seems to be less effective. Daily colchicine is reasonably effective in preventing flares while ULT is titrated.[58,59] In a patient with CKD stage 3 or greater, NSAIDs should be avoided, and colchicine should be dose-reduced or not used at all because of concerns of toxicity.[38] As discussed above, caution must be exercised as drug-drug interactions can occur when colchicine is used in combination with CYP3A4 or P-glycoprotein inhibitors, particularly in the setting of CKD. Reversible but significant painful axonal neurotoxicity and vacuolar myopathy have been well described.

There are strong data demonstrating that IL-1 inhibition provides effective anti-inflammatory prophylaxis. This prophylactic strategy may be particularly helpful in patients who have contraindications to colchicine and NSAIDs, but it is not currently FDA approved and is expensive.

WHEN TO CONSIDER AGGRESSIVE URATE-LOWERING THERAPY

Pegloticase is a recombinant mammalian uricase conjugated to polyethylene glycol (PEG) used to dramatically lower the SUA and treat refractory gout.[35,60] There are several situations in which gout patients should be considered for pegloticase administration. If a patient fails to reach serum urate goal on maximally tolerated ULT, then pegloticase should be considered.[49] Pegloticase should also be considered if there are contraindications to the administration or optimization of oral urate-lowering agents. As outlined in **Fig. 1**, pegloticase should also be considered if urgent resolution of tophi deposition is needed or desired by the patient (eg,

5/2014 SUA 10.1 on febuxostat 80 mg (allergic to allopurinol); creatinine 2.4. attacks every few weeks

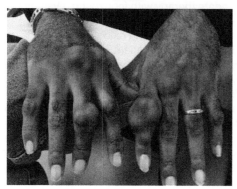

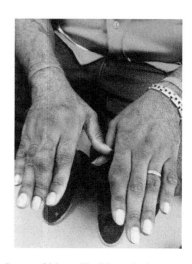

9 mo of biweekly IV pegloticase
SUA <0.2 mg/dL. No attacks in >3 mo

Fig. 2. Efficacy of dramatic lowering of serum urate on tophi. IV, intravenous.

nonhealing infected tophus, impending organ transplantation, if the patient is unable to perform daily activities owing to tophus deposition, or if there is a particularly large or burdensome tophus deposition that would likely require years to dissolve with the use of traditional ULT).[49,61,62] Pegloticase is administered every 2 to 3 weeks (the label states every 2 weeks) by intravenous infusion for several months; the duration is based on goals of therapy and the patient's response. Pegloticase can lower the SUA to almost unmeasurable levels, and shrinkage of palpable tophi and improved function of seriously involved joints can be demonstrated over several months (**Fig. 2**). With the dramatic drop in the SUA (often <0.2 mg/dL) with this drug during therapy, mobilization flares are expected and may be severe before the deposits are gone and the flares cease to occur. However, in clinical trials, ~60% of patients rapidly developed high-titer drug neutralizing antibodies to the PEG. The drug had limited (but measurable) benefit in these "nonresponding" patients, and those with neutralizing antibodies were more likely to have infusion reactions. Thus, the drug should be discontinued in patients who have 2 consecutive preinfusion SUA levels of greater than 6 mg/dL. Several recent observational studies suggest that coadministration with methotrexate, mycophenolate, or other immunosuppressive medications may prevent the development of these anti-PEG antibodies. A randomized prospective trial has recently been completed, and initial results indicate that immunosuppression with methotrexate is quite effective at preventing the occurrence of drug resistance. After a successful course of pegloticase therapy, it is discontinued, and traditional ULT is resumed, with the goal of keeping the SUA to less than 6 mg/dL to prevent recurrence of hyperuricemia with urate deposition.

DISCLOSURE

S.F. Keller has nothing to disclose. B.F. Mandell: Clinical Investigator: Horizon Pharmaceuticals; Consultant: Horizon Pharmaceuticals, Sobi Pharmaceuticals.

REFERENCES

1. Chen-Xu M, Yokose C, Rai SK, et al. Contemporary prevalence of gout and hyper-uricemia in the United States and decadal trends: the National Health and Nutrition Examination Survey, 2007–2016. Arthritis Rheumatol 2019;71(6):991–9.
2. Janssens HJEM, Fransen J, Van De Lisdonk EH, et al. A diagnostic rule for acute gouty arthritis in primary care without joint fluid analysis. Arch Intern Med 2010; 170(13):1120–6.
3. Greenspan A, Gershwin ME. Metabolic, endocrine, and crystal deposition arthropathies. In: Greenspan A, Gershwin ME, editors. Imaging in rheumatology: a clinical approach. 1st edition. Wolters Kluwer Health; 2018. p. 269–309.
4. Brower AC, Flemming DJ. Gout. In: Brower AC, Flemming DJ, editors. Arthritis in black and white. 3rd edition. Elsevier Health Sciences; 2012. p. 293–308.
5. Samuels JTK. Basic ultrasound pathology. In: Kohler MJ, editor. Musculoskeletal ultrasound in rheumatology review. 1st edition. Springer International Publishing; 2016. p. 23–55.
6. O'Neill JO. Crystal-related disease. In: O'Neill J, editor. Essential imaging in rheumatology. Springer; 2015. p. 213–32.
7. Gamala M, Jacobs JWG, van Lear JM. The diagnostic performance of dual energy CT for diagnosing gout: a systematic literature review and meta-analysis. Rheumatol 2019;58(12):2117–21.
8. FitzGerald JD, Dalbeth N, Mikuls T, et al. American College of Rheumatology Guideline for the management of gout. Arthritis Care Res (Hoboken) 2020; 72(6):744–60.
9. Richette P, Doherty M, Pascual E, et al. 2016 updated EULAR evidence-based recommendations for the management of gout. Ann Rheum Dis 2017;76(1): 29–42.
10. Terkeltaub RA. Clinical practice. Gout. N Engl J Med 2003;349(17):1647–55.
11. Roddy E, Clarkson K, Blagojevic-Bucknall M, et al. Open-label randomised pragmatic trial (CONTACT) comparing naproxen and low-dose colchicine for the treatment of gout flares in primary care. Ann Rheum Dis 2020;79(2):276–84.
12. Schumacher HR, Berger MF, Li-Yu J, et al. Efficacy and tolerability of celecoxib in the treatment of acute gouty arthritis: a randomized controlled trial. J Rheumatol 2012;39(9):1859–66.
13. Kuo C-F, Grainge MJ, Mallen C, et al. Comorbidities in patients with gout prior to and following diagnosis: case-control study. Ann Rheum Dis 2016;75(1):210–7.
14. Terkeltaub RA, Furst DE, Bennett K, et al. High versus low dosing of oral colchicine for early acute gout flare: twenty-four-hour outcome of the first multicenter, randomized, double-blind, placebo-controlled, parallel-group, dose-comparison colchicine study. Arthritis Rheum 2010;62(4):1060–8.
15. Terkeltaub R. Update on gout: new therapeutic strategies and options. Nat Rev Rheumatol 2010;6(1):30–8.
16. Slobodnick A, Shah B, Pillinger MH, et al. Colchicine: old and new. Am J Med 2015;128(5):461–70.
17. Janssens EM, Janssen M, van de Lisdonk EH, et al. Use of oral prednisolone or naproxen for the treatment of gout arthritis: a double-blind. randomised equivalence trial, 371, 2008. www.thelancet.com.
18. Man CY, Cheung ITF, Cameron PA, et al. Comparison of oral prednisolone/paracetamol and oral indomethacin/paracetamol combination therapy in the treatment of acute goutlike arthritis: a double-blind, randomized, controlled trial. Ann Emerg Med 2007;49(5):670–7.

19. Elliott EI, Sutterwala FS. Initiation and perpetuation of NLRP3 inflammasome activation and assembly. Immunol Rev 2015;265(1):35–52.

20. Martinon F, Pétrilli V, Mayor A, et al. Gout-associated uric acid crystals activate the NALP3 inflammasome. Nature 2006;440(7081):237–41.

21. Fisher CJ, Dhainaut JF, Opal SM, et al. Recombinant human interleukin 1 receptor antagonist in the treatment of patients with sepsis syndrome. Results from a randomized, double-blind, placebo-controlled trial. Phase III rhIL-1ra Sepsis Syndrome Study Group. JAMA 1994;271(23):1836–43.

22. Liew JW, Gardner GC. Use of anakinra in hospitalized patients with crystal-associated arthritis. J Rheumatol 2019;46(10):1345–9.

23. Balasubramaniam G, Parker T, Turner D, et al. Feasibility randomised multicentre, double-blind, double-dummy controlled trial of anakinra, an interleukin-1 receptor antagonist versus intramuscular methylprednisolone for acute gout attacks in patients with chronic kidney disease (ASGARD): protocol study. BMJ Open 2017;7(9).

24. Mandell BF. Clinical manifestations of hyperuricemia and gout. Cleve Clin J Med 2008;75(SUPPL.5):5–8.

25. Dalbeth N, Phipps-Green A, Frampton C, et al. Relationship between serum urate concentration and clinically evident incident gout: an individual participant data analysis. Ann Rheum Dis 2018 Jul;77(7):1048–52.

26. Dalbeth N, Chen P, White M, et al. Impact of bariatric surgery on serum urate targets in people with morbid obesity and diabetes: a prospective longitudinal study. Ann Rheum Dis 2014;73(5):797–802.

27. Choi HK, Atkinson K, Karlson EW, et al. Purine-rich foods, daily and protein intake, and the risk of gout in men. N Engl J Med 2004;350(11):1093–103.

28. Choi HK, Atkinson K, Karlson EW, et al. Alcohol intake and risk of incident gout in men: a prospective study. Lancet 2004;363(9417):1277–81.

29. Choi HK, Curhan G. Soft drinks, fructose consumption, and the risk of gout in men: prospective cohort study. BMJ 2008;336(7639):309–12.

30. Schumacher HR. The pathogenesis of gout. Cleve Clin J Med 2008; 75(SUPPL.5):2–4.

31. Shoji A, Yamanaka H, Kamatani N. A retrospective study of the relationship between serum urate level and recurrent attacks of gouty arthritis: evidence for reduction of recurrent gouty arthritis with antihyperuricemic therapy. Arthritis Care Res (Hoboken) 2004;51(3):321–5.

32. Mandell BF. Hyperuricemia and gout: a reign of complacency. Cleve Clin J Med 2002;69(8):589–93.

33. Yamanaka H, Togashi R, Hakoda M, et al. Optimal range of serum urate concentrations to minimize risk of gouty attacks during anti-hyperuricemic treatment. In: Advances in Experimental medicine and Biology. Vol 431. Adv Exp Med Biol; 1998:13-18.

34. O'Dell J, Neogi T, Pillinger M, et al. Urate lowering therapy in the treatment of gout: a multicenter, randomized, double-blind comparison of allopurinol and febuxostat using a treat-to-target strategy. Arthritis Rheumatol 2021;73(suppl 10).

35. Sundy JS, Baraf HSB, Yood RA, et al. Efficacy and tolerability of pegloticase for the treatment of chronic gout in patients refractory to conventional treatment: two randomized controlled trials. J Am Med Assoc 2011;306(7):711–20.

36. Stamp LK, Frampton C, Morillon MB, et al. Association between serum urate and flares in people with gout and evidence for surrogate status: a secondary analysis of two randomised controlled trials. Lancet Rheumatol 2022;4:e53–60.

37. Edwards NL. The role of hyperuricemia and gout in kidney and cardiovascular disease. Cleve Clin J Med 2008;75(SUPPL.5):13–6.
38. Vargas-Santos AB, Neogi T. Management of gout and hyperuricemia in CKD. Am J Kidney Dis 2017;70(3):422–39.
39. Santhosh Pai BH, Swarnalatha G, Ram R, et al. Allopurinol for prevention of progression of kidney disease with hyperuricemia. Indian J Nephrol 2013;23(4): 280–6.
40. Levy GD, Rashid N, Niu F, et al. Effect of urate-lowering therapies on renal disease progression in patients with hyperuricemia. J Rheumatol 2014;41(5): 955–62.
41. Whelton A, MacDonald PA, Zhao L, et al. Renal function in gout: long-term treatment effects of febuxostat. J Clin Rheumatol 2011;17(1):7–13.
42. Tomita M, Mizuno S, Yamanaka H, et al. Does hyperuricemia affect mortality? A prospective cohort study of Japanese male workers. J Epidemiol 2000;10(6): 403–9.
43. Iseki K, Ikemiya Y, Inoue T, et al. Significance of hyperuricemia as a risk factor for developing ESRD in a screened cohort. Am J Kidney Dis 2004;44(4):642–50.
44. Feig DI. Urate-lowering therapy and chronic kidney disease progression. N Engl J Med 2020;382(26):2567–8.
45. Ioachimescu AG, Brennan DM, Hoar BM, et al. Serum uric acid is an independent predictor of all-cause mortality in patients at high risk of cardiovascular disease: a Preventive Cardiology Information System (PreCIS) database cohort study. Arthritis Rheum 2008;58(2):623–30.
46. Pérez Ruiz F, Richette P, Stack AG, et al. Failure to reach uric acid target of <0.36 mmol/L in hyperuricaemia of gout is associated with elevated total and cardiovascular mortality. RMD Open 2019;5(2).
47. Zuo T, Liu X, Jiang L, et al. Hyperuricemia and coronary heart disease mortality: a meta-analysis of prospective cohort studies. BMC Cardiovasc Disord 2016; 16(1):207.
48. Chen J-H, Chuang S-Y, Chen H-J, et al. Serum uric acid level as an independent risk factor for all-cause, cardiovascular, and ischemic stroke mortality: a Chinese cohort study. Arthritis Rheum 2009;61(2):225–32.
49. Pillinger MH, Mandell BF. Therapeutic approaches in the treatment of gout. Semin Arthritis Rheum 2020;50(3):S24–30.
50. Stamp LK, Chapman PT, Barclay ML, et al. A randomised controlled trial of the efficacy and safety of allopurinol dose escalation to achieve target serum urate in people with gout. Ann Rheum Dis 2017;76(9):1522–8.
51. Yang CY, Chen CH, Deng ST, et al. Allopurinol use and risk of fatal hypersensitivity reactions: a nationwide population-based study in Taiwan. JAMA Intern Med 2015;175(9):1550–7.
52. Keller SF, Lu N, Blumenthal KG, et al. Racial/ethnic variation and risk factors for allopurinol-associated severe cutaneous adverse reactions: a cohort study. Ann Rheum Dis 2018;77(8):1187–93.
53. Stamp LK, Taylor WJ, Jones PB, et al. Starting dose is a risk factor for allopurinol hypersensitivity syndrome: a proposed safe starting dose of allopurinol. Arthritis Rheum 2012;64(8):2529–36.
54. Becker MA, Schumacher HR, Wortmann RL, et al. Febuxostat compared with allopurinol in patients with hyperuricemia and gout. N Engl J Med 2005; 353(23):2450–61.
55. White WB, Saag KG, Becker MA, et al. Cardiovascular safety of febuxostat or allopurinol in patients with gout. N Engl J Med 2018;378(13):1200–10.

56. Mackenzie IS, Ford I, Nuki G, et al. Long-term cardiovascular safety of febuxostat compared with allopurinol in patients with gout (FAST): a multicentre, prospective, randomised, open-label, non-inferiority trial. Lancet 2020. https://doi.org/10.1016/S0140-6736(20)32234-0.

57. Tausche A-K, Alten R, Dalbeth N, et al. Lesinurad monotherapy in gout patients intolerant to a xanthine oxidase inhibitor: a 6 month phase 3 clinical trial and extension study. Rheumatology (Oxford) 2017;56(12):2170–8.

58. Borstad GC, Bryant LR, Abel MP, et al. Colchicine for prophylaxis of acute flares when initiating allopurinol for chronic gouty arthritis. J Rheumatol 2004;31(12):2429–32.

59. Paulus HE, Schlosstein LH, Godfrey RG, et al. Prophylactic colchicine therapy of intercritical gout. A placebo-controlled study of probenecid-treated patients. Arthritis Rheum 1974;17(5):609–14.

60. Baraf HSB, Becker MA, Gutierrez-Urena SR, et al. Tophus burden reduction with pegloticase: results from phase 3 randomized trials and open-label extension in patients with chronic gout refractory to conventional therapy. Arthritis Res Ther 2013;15(5).

61. Mandell BF, Yeo AE, Lipsky PE. Tophus resolution in patients with chronic refractory gout who have persistent urate-lowering responses to pegloticase. Arthritis Res Ther 2018;20(1).

62. Strand V, Khanna D, Singh JA, et al. Improved health-related quality of life and physical function in patients with refractory chronic gout following treatment with pegloticase: evidence from phase III randomized controlled trials. J Rheumatol 2012;39(7):1450–7.

Update on the Treatment of Giant Cell Arteritis and Polymyalgia Rheumatica

Sarah El Chami, MBBS[a], Jason M. Springer, MD, MS[b],*

KEYWORDS

- Giant cell arteritis • Polymyalgia rheumatica • Large vessel vasculitis
- Temporal arteritis • Tocilizumab

KEY POINTS

- Frequently, polymyalgia rheumatica (PMR) and giant cell arteritis (GCA) overlap in the same patient. PMR may be a forme fruste of GCA.
- Although the cranial phenotype is the most common phenotype of GCA, other phenotypes exist and need to be recognized.
- Temporal artery biopsy remains the gold standard for diagnosis of GCA with new roles for cranial imaging in diagnosis and management.
- Screening for large vessel involvement should be performed in all cases of GCA, as it is often asymptomatic and associated with a poorer prognosis.
- Glucocorticoids remain the cornerstone of treatment in both GCA and PMR with an emerging role for steroid-sparing agents. The results of a randomized controlled trial demonstrated tocilizumab to be effective in the treatment of GCA.

GIANT CELL ARTERITIS

Introduction

Giant cell arteritis (GCA) is the most common form of primary systemic vasculitis in North America with an incidence greater than 17 per 100,000 in those older than 50 years. This disease almost always affects individuals older than 50 years with a peak incidence in the 70- to 79-year age group. The incidence of GCA increases with latitude in the Northern hemisphere. GCA much more commonly affects women (3:1 ratio of women to men) and Caucasian populations, with a low incidence in black, Hispanic, and Asian populations.[1] Early recognition and prompt treatment of GCA is crucial to prevent catastrophic ischemic complications.

This article originally appeared in the Medical Clinics of North America, Volume 105, Issue 2, March 2021.

[a] The University of Kansas Health System, 4000 Cambridge Street, MS 2026, Kansas City, KS 66160, USA; [b] Vanderbilt University Medical Center 1161 21st Avenue South, T-3113 Medical Center North Nashville, TN 37232-2681, USA

* Corresponding author.

E-mail address: jason.springer@vumc.org

Rheum Dis Clin N Am 48 (2022) 493–506
https://doi.org/10.1016/j.rdc.2022.02.007
0889-857X/22/© 2022 Elsevier Inc. All rights reserved.

Clinical Phenotypes

de Boysson and colleagues[2] identified 4 clinical patterns of GCA in a retrospective analysis of 693 patients with GCA. The cranial phenotype, constituting 80% of cases, presents with temporal headache, temporal artery abnormalities (eg, tenderness or decrease pulsation), jaw/tongue claudication, and/or scalp tenderness. This phenotype has the highest risk of early ocular ischemic events. The presence of intracranial involvement is not characteristic of GCA and should prompt consideration of an alternative diagnosis. Another pattern includes large vessel involvement (ie, the aorta and its major branches), present in 9% of cases. Common clinical features include limb claudication, asymmetric peripheral pulses, lightheadedness, hypertension, subclavian steal syndrome, aortic aneurysms, and aortic valve regurgitation. The third group, representing about 9% of patients, presents with fever of unknown origin and elevated inflammatory markers. The final group includes patients who clinically seem to have isolated polymyalgia rheumatica (PMR) but have evidence of asymptomatic vasculitis on arterial biopsy or imaging. However, it is recognized that these phenotypes are not mutually exclusive, with a subset of patients demonstrating overlapping clinical features.

Diagnosis

The diagnosis of GCA can be confirmed by either a temporal artery biopsy (TAB) or imaging showing arteritis. However, both modalities can have false-negative results rendering it challenging to completely rule out the disease, especially when a high index of suspicion exists.

Temporal artery biopsy

Classic histologic changes include chronic granulomatous inflammation generally concentrated at the level of the internal elastic lamina, intimal hyperplasia, giant cell formation, fragmentation of the internal elastic lamina, and vessel wall necrosis. The inflammatory infiltrate consists of epithelioid histiocytes, multinucleated giant cells, T lymphocytes, and macrophages. The inflammatory infiltrate is thought to initially enter through the vasa vasorum and progress from the adventitia inwardly within the arterial wall.[3] Inflammation can progress in a patchy distribution along the artery, leaving some areas of the artery unaffected. Within this age group, polyarteritis nodosa– and antineutrophil cytoplasmic antibody–associated vasculitis can also cause inflammatory changes of the temporal artery or surrounding vessels, mimicking GCA pathologically. A fibrotic pattern, reflecting damage from prior inflammation, can be difficult to differentiate from normal arterial aging of the temporal artery.[4]

The temporal artery biopsy has been considered by many as the gold standard for diagnosis. However, because of the patchy nature of the inflammatory infiltrate, a negative biopsy does not rule out the disease. The sensitivity can vary depending on the center and prevalence of disease. One study showed that 87% of patients with negative biopsies were continued on glucocorticoids based on clinical concerns for GCA.[5] In the presence of a very high clinical suspicion, histologic confirmation may not be needed. The authors recommend obtaining temporal artery biopsies in patients with cranial symptoms suspicious for GCA when there is diagnostic uncertainty and/or an atypical presentation.

The length and laterality of the temporal artery biopsy is another important consideration. Postfixation lengths of at least 2 cm are ideal but can be difficult to achieve in clinical practice. A 2006 retrospective review of more than 1000 temporal artery biopsies suggested that even a 0.5 cm biopsy can be adequate.[6] The symptomatic side of the head should be the target of the biopsy. Obtaining bilateral temporal artery biopsies can increase the yield modestly. Bilateral temporal artery biopsies have been estimated to have a discordance rate of 4.4%.[7] Based on the expertise of the center a contralateral biopsy could be considered, either done after a negative finding on frozen section of the initial biopsy or simultaneously. Procedural complications are rare but can include infection, nerve damage, bleeding, and scarring. Obtaining a TAB should be done as soon as feasible; however, several studies have shown that a biopsy remains useful even after several weeks of treatment. TAB results can change after initiation of glucocorticoid therapy showing atypical features or healing arteritis.[8]

Imaging
Cranial imaging There is limited evidence supporting the use of head MRI for the diagnosis of GCA with cranial artery involvement. Bley and colleagues[9] have shown high-resolution contrast-enhanced MRI of the cranial arteries had a sensitivity of 81% and specificity of 97% based on the 1990 American College of Rheumatology (ACR) criteria (91% sensitivity and 73% specificity based on histologically confirmed cases). However, these results depend on the strength of the magnet (3 T preferred) and the protocol used.[10,11] The sensitivity is dramatically reduced when imaging is done after 5 to 10 days of starting glucocorticoids.[9,12]

Color doppler ultrasonography (CDUS) is a noninvasive means to assess cranial arteries in GCA. The presence of a halo sign, stenosis, or occlusion of the common temporal artery, its branches, or the facial artery can be used to support the diagnosis of GCA. However, the utility of CDUS for diagnosis of GCA highly depends on the experience of the ultrasonographer. In a large, prospective, multicenter study including 381 patients with newly suspected GCA, a training program for CDUS of the temporal and axillary arteries was implemented.[13] Using the 1990 ACR classification criteria and final clinical diagnosis, CDUS had a higher sensitivity (54% [95% confidence interval [CI] 48%–60%] vs 39% [95% CI 33%–46%]) but lower specificity (81% [95% CI 73%–88%] vs 100% [95% CI 97%–100%]) compared with temporal artery biopsy. Using an approach of first evaluating with CDUS followed by a temporal artery biopsy in those with negative CDUS, the sensitivity increased to 65% while maintaining a specificity of 81%, reducing the need for biopsies by 43%. Inter-rater agreement for CDUS was moderate (r = 0.69, 95% CI 0.48–0.75), but similar to the inter-rater agreement for pathology assessment (r = 0.62, 95% CI 0.49–0.76). Of note, CDUS was done within 7 days of starting glucocorticoids.

The sensitivity and specificity of high-resolution MRI and CDUS for diagnosis of cranial GCA seems to be comparable.[14] However, the utility of these imaging modalities depend on the availability of appropriate equipment, protocols, and center experience with these modalities. Thus, for many centers TAB remains the preferred diagnostic modality for patients with suspected GCA presenting with cranial manifestations.

Large vessel imaging GCA is known to involve a larger network of vessels outside of cranial vasculature (ie, the aorta and major branches). Large-artery complications, including thoracic or abdominal aortic aneurysm and/or dissection, are associated with a high mortality.[15] This mandates the need for early detection through screening with appropriate follow-up. The presence of physical examination abnormalities in patients with established large vessel vasculitis (eg, absent carotid or radial pulse, carotid or subclavian bruit, or systolic blood pressure difference of more than 10 mm Hg) has a sensitivity as low as 14% in detecting arterial abnormalities in large vessel vasculitis and should be supplemented by imaging.[16] The estimated rate of asymptomatic large vessel involvement is 30% to 80%.[17] Conventional angiography has been largely replaced by noninvasive imaging for screening purposes but still appropriate for interventional procedures in cases of critical stenosis or aneurysmal dilation. Otherwise, there is not a clearly preferred modality for the evaluation of extra-cranial large vessel involvement.

Computed tomography angiography (CTA), PET/CT, and MR angiography (MRA) are all noninvasive modalities that can be used either for diagnosis or follow-up monitoring of large vessel disease (**Fig. 1**). CTA offers the advantage of giving a high degree of anatomic detail, but the radiation exposure may make this a less desirable option for long-term follow-up. PET/CT has the highest sensitivity of picking up aortic

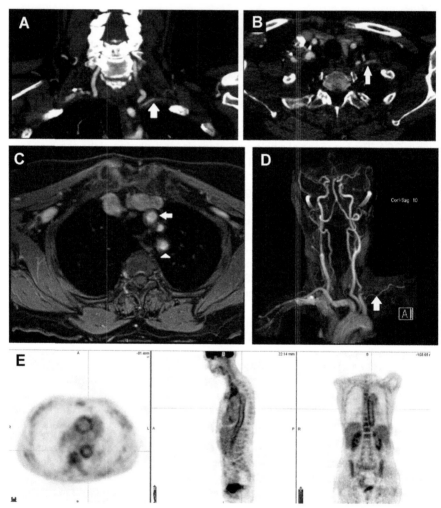

Fig. 1. A 64-year-old woman with predominantly large vessel involvement. CTA with and without contrast showing abrupt occlusion of the left subclavian artery (*arrow* in *A* and *B*). High-resolution MRI of the head and neck with and without contrast demonstrates mural thickening and contrast enhancement of the left brachiocephalic artery (*arrow* in *C*) and left subclavian artery (*arrowhead* in *C*). Left subclavian artery vessel wall occlusion with collateral formation (*arrow* in *D*). (*E*) Thoracic and abdominal aortitis in a separate patient as imaged by PET/CT.

inflammation, making it a good option to assist with the diagnosis of GCA; however, the uptake is not specific for GCA. Forms of secondary large vessel vasculitis (eg, syphilis, tuberculosis, sarcoidosis) and atherosclerosis can all mimic GCA on PET/CT. The high cost, limited accessibility, and radiation exposure make PET/CT a less desirable option for long-term follow-up of patients with large vessel involvement. MRA offers the advantage of good visualization of the arterial wall for inflammatory changes. Because of the lack of radiation exposure, it may be a preferable option for follow-up imaging for patients with known large vessel disease in centers with accessible equipment (3T magnet preferred) and experienced radiologists. The use of gadolinium-based contrast agents in patients with estimated glomerular filtration rate less than 30 mL/min/1.73 m^2 is associated with the development of nephrogenic systemic fibrosis. Although the use of newer contrast agents has substantially decreased that risk, clinician should still use caution in patient with chronic renal insufficiency.

CDUS can provide information on some of the more superficial large arteries (eg, subclavian, axillary, abdominal aortic, and common femoral arteries), with the highest sensitivity in the subclavian and axillary arteries.[18] However, in this setting CDUS has multiple limitations including inability to visualize many large arteries, the time-intensive nature of examination, and the dependence of the expertise of the sonographer. CDUS may be a valuable alternative in patients unable or with contraindications to other imaging modalities (eg, chronic renal insufficiency).

The choice and frequency of large vessel imaging depend on the clinical setting. In patients with known large vessel involvement, follow-up imaging is recommended. Although the optimal frequency is not established, the authors recommend obtaining imaging every 6 to 12 months until vascular stability has been established. In patients without known large vessel involvement, baseline imaging is recommended with follow-up imaging based on suspicious clinical features (eg, extremity claudication, unexplained elevations in inflammatory markers, and asymmetrical pulses and/or blood pressure). Given the known increased mortality of thoracic aortic aneurysm and dissection, yearly echocardiogram and chest radiograph to screen for these potential complications should be considered in all patients with GCA if more advanced imaging is not already being done (**Table 1**).

Glucocorticoid Effects on Diagnostic Modalities

Although glucocorticoids can decrease the sensitivity of many diagnostic modalities, prompt treatment should not be withheld in those with a high clinical suspicion while waiting for completion of diagnostic testing. A large retrospective study that included 535 patients with GCA demonstrated a similar rate of positive biopsies in untreated and treated patients even after 14 days of therapy.[8] Glucocorticoids can quickly affect finding on imaging. Thus, noninvasive imaging modalities are best done within 4 to 5 days of starting glucocorticoids to pick up acute inflammation.[12,19]

Laboratory studies

Unfortunately, there are no biomarkers that are specific to the diagnosis of GCA. Erythrocyte sedimentation rate (ESR) and C-reactive protein (CRP) are typically elevated but not specific. In a large retrospective study that included 177 patients with biopsy proven GCA, elevated CRP and elevated ESR provided a sensitivity of 87% and 84%, respectively, for a positive TAB. On the other hand, the presence of normal ESR and CRP did not exclude the diagnosis of GCA, as 4% of these patients had normal ESR and CRP.[20] Patients can also have anemia of chronic disease or elevated alkaline phosphatase.

Table 1
Comparison of noninvasive diagnostic imaging modalities in giant cell arteritis

Imaging Modality	Advantages	Disadvantages
CTA	• Noninvasive • Accessible • High anatomic detail • Information on vessel wall inflammation	• Radiation exposure • Need for iodinated contrast • Limitation in use with patient with renal insufficiency
PET/CT	• Noninvasive • Highest sensitivity for vessel wall inflammation	• High cost • Accessibility • Radiation exposure • Uptake is not specific for vasculitis
MRI/MRA Cranial MRI Large vessel MRA	• Noninvasive • No radiation exposure • Evaluates both vessel wall inflammation and structure	• High cost • Limited use in those with renal impairment or metal implants • Difficult in claustrophobic patients • Need for radiologist expertise
CDUS Cranial Large vessel	• Noninvasive • No radiation exposure • Low cost • Evaluates both vessel wall structure and inflammation • Limited evaluation of large vessels	• Operator dependent • Not ideal for visualization of thoracic aorta
Echocardiogram	• Noninvasive • No radiation exposure • Low cost • Screening for ascending thoracic aortic aneurysms	• Limited to evaluation of the aortic root • Advanced imaging required if abnormal
Chest radiograph	• Noninvasive • Minimal radiation exposure • Low cost • Screening for thoracic aortic aneurysm	• No detail on vessel wall. • Limited to thoracic aorta. • Advanced imaging required if abnormal • Findings might not correlate with final diagnosis

Treatment of Giant Cell Arteritis

Glucocorticoids

Prompt initiation of glucocorticoids is required to prevent the dreaded ischemic complications including irreversible vision loss. There are conflicting reports behind the use of intravenous, "pulse" glucocorticoids. A double-blinded placebo-controlled study including 27 patients with biopsy-proven GCA showed induction with methylprednisolone, 15 mg/kg/d, for 3 days permits a shorter course of therapy, higher sustained remission, and lower median dose of steroids compared with placebo.[21] On the other hand, another randomized multicenter prospective trial showed no added benefit of using a single infusion of 240 mg intravenous methylprednisolone, a much lower dose, in terms of time needed to taper off glucocorticoids, mean cumulative prednisone dose, or steroid-related side effects.[22] In the setting of vision loss due to ischemic complications the authors recommend the use of intravenous pulse glucocorticoids followed by oral, as endorsed by both the European League Against Rheumatism and the British Society for Rheumatology.[23,24] Vision loss in patients with GCA is most commonly from arteritic anterior ischemic optic neuropathy (AAION), which, compared with nonarteritic anterior ischemic optic neuropathy, rarely improves. AAION can involve the contralateral eye. Hence, it is imperative to promptly start glucocorticoid treatment to prevent contralateral eye involvement.

Patients require initial high doses of oral glucocorticoids, typically followed by a prolonged taper with a mean duration of treatment ranging from 31 to 40 months.[25,26] Alternate day dosing of oral glucocorticoids is not recommended, as patients can become symptomatic on days not taken.[27] The frequent relapses and glucocorticoid-related side effects with glucocorticoid monotherapy has led to the investigation of other immunosuppressive medications to limit the cumulative glucocorticoid exposure.

Tocilizumab

A phase II randomized, double-blind, placebo-controlled trial supported intravenous tocilizumab for the treatment of GCA. Patients in the treatment group received 13 infusions of intravenous tocilizumab (8 mg/kg, once monthly) along with a standardized prednisone taper. Eighty percent of patients in the tocilizumab group tapered prednisone to 0 mg by 52 weeks compared with 20% of patients in the placebo group, and the cumulative dose of prednisone was significantly higher in the placebo group at week 52 (67 mg/kg difference). There were no infusion-related adverse events, and the overall adverse events were similar in the 2 groups. Serious adverse events were higher in the placebo group. Neutropenia was an adverse event noted in tocilizumab group (4 patients) but not in the placebo group. No relapses occurred in the tocilizumab group by 52 weeks.[28]

In a phase III randomized double-blinded placebo-controlled trial 251 patients with GCA were randomized to 4 groups: 2 arms receiving tocilizumab, 162 mg, weekly or every other week injections combined with a 26-week prednisone taper and 2 placebo groups that received a prednisone taper over 26 or 52 weeks. The tocilizumab groups had a superior glucocorticoid-free remission compared with either of the control groups. Neutropenia was slightly higher in the tocilizumab group; otherwise, the rate of adverse events did not differ between the 2 groups. There were no bowel wall perforations seen; however, patients at higher risk (ie, prior history of diverticulitis or gastrointestinal perforation) were excluded given previous data of increased risk of lower gastrointestinal perforation with tocilizumab treatment in patients with rheumatoid arthritis.[29] Patients in the placebo groups received almost double the cumulative glucocorticoid dose. Weekly tocilizumab resulted in greater disease control compared with every other week; however, both tocilizumab groups fared better than placebo groups.[30] There have been isolated reports of patients found to have active arteritis by biopsy despite apparent good disease control with tocilizumab, which has raised concern by some that tocilizumab may be blunting clinical symptoms without fully controlling the underlying disease process.[31]

The optimal duration of tocilizumab treatment remains unknown. A 2-year extension of the phase III trial demonstrated that a significant number of patients relapsed after stopping tocilizumab after 1 year. However, patients who developed a relapse responded to retreatment with tocilizumab.[32] Based on these data, the authors suggest continuing tocilizumab treatment of at least 2 years. This decision needs to be determined on case-by-case basis while weighing risks versus benefits of continued therapy in individual patients.

Although both intravenous and subcutaneous routes of treatment with tocilizumab can be effective treatment options, there are important points to keep in mind before initiating treatment. Tocilizumab has a blunting effect on the acute phase response of the liver making the sedimentation rate and CRP less reliable biomarkers. A careful assessment of the risks and benefits should be exercised in patients at higher risk of bowel perforation (eg, prior history of diverticulitis or gastrointestinal perforation). Many patients can develop significant hypercholesterolemia with a mean increase in nonfasting total cholesterol level by 35 mg/dL at 12 months; however, subsequent cholesterol levels generally remain stable. The increase in the cholesterol level is not paralleled with an increase in cardiovascular events.[33] Tocilizumab prescribing information recommend assessing lipid parameters approximately 4 to 8 weeks following initiation of therapy, then at approximately 24-week intervals.

Other agents

There are conflicting reports regarding the use of methotrexate (MTX) in the treatment of GCA. Three randomized double-blind placebo-controlled trials were published on treatment with methotrexate (MTX) in GCA between 2001 and 2002.[34–36] The differences in results may be explained by the duration of MTX treatment, with the steroid-sparing effects seen most prominently in those treated for at least 24 months (compared with 12–17 months). A meta-analysis of the abovementioned trials concluded the addition of MTX reduces the risk of first relapse by 35% and that of second relapse by 51%. This was associated with a reduction in cumulative prednisone dose and a higher probability of achieving sustained remission.[37] The authors recommend the use of MTX as a second-line option in those patients with relapsing/refractory disease or with contraindications to tocilizumab, such as hypersensitivity reactions to tocilizumab or increased risk of GI perforation, at doses of at least 15 mg weekly (oral or subcutaneous) for at least 24 months.

Abatacept, a cytotoxic T-lymphocyte antigen 4 mimetic, and ustekinumab, an interleukin-12 (IL-12) and IL-23 inhibitor, have shown promising results in small clinical trials. Larger trials are warranted to further evaluate the effectiveness of both those treatments in GCA. Tumor necrosis factor (TNF) inhibitors have not been shown to have a benefit in GCA.

Adjunctive therapies

There have been conflicting reports regarding the use of low-dose aspirin as a preventative measure against arterial complications in GCA. A retrospective study by Salvarani and colleagues[38] showed patients who were on antiplatelet or anticoagulation therapy had higher risk of developing cranial ischemic events. This may reflect the higher propensity for patients with more cardiovascular risk factor to receive aspirin.

Another retrospective study showed that low-dose aspirin decreases the rate of visual loss and cerebrovascular accidents in patients with GCA by 5 times.[39] Although there are no randomized trials addressing the use of aspirin in GCA, the authors recommend use of low-dose aspirin in patients without contraindications, such as the use of other antiplatelet or anticoagulant drugs. A retrospective study published in 2007 did not find evidence of statin benefit in decreasing the incidence of ischemic complications or disease outcome.[40]

POLYMYALGIA RHEUMATICA

PMR is also more common in white individuals of northern European background, women and older individual, with a mean age around 74 years. Individuals of Asian, African American, American Indian, or other races were much less likely to be affected.[41] PMR is 2 to 3 times more common than GCA.[1,42] It is estimated that 40% to 60% of patients with GCA have PMR. Only 16% to 21% of patients with PMR have GCA, although large vessel involvement may be underrecognized.[41]

Diagnosis

The diagnosis of PMR is largely clinical. The diagnosis of PMR should be suspected in individuals older than 50 years who present with pain and stiffness of the neck, shoulders or pelvic girdle areas, morning stiffness, and/or elevated inflammatory markers. The disease should be considered when symptom duration lasts more than 2 weeks. Prompt response to moderate doses of glucocorticoids (15–25 mg daily of prednisone or its equivalent) further supports the diagnosis. Common mimics to exclude include statin-induced myopathy, infections, malignancy, mechanical shoulder/hip pathology, inflammatory myopathies, fibromyalgia, hypothyroidism, GCA, and rheumatoid arthritis. In addition to a comprehensive physical examination, review of systems, and medication review, the authors recommend, the basic workup to include a complete blood count with differential, comprehensive metabolic panel, sedimentation rate, CRP, rheumatoid factor, anti-CCP, thyroid-stimulating hormone, serum/urine protein electrophoresis, creatine kinase, and infectious evaluation as appropriate. The association of PMR with distal extremity inflammatory arthritis has been described in the literature in up to 50% of the patients in some reports. Wrist synovitis, when present, can present with symptoms of carpal tunnel syndrome. The presence of significant distal inflammatory arthritis, especially with ankle and metatarsophalangeal joint involvement, should prompt consideration of an alternative diagnosis. In a similar fashion, in patients with PMR who are asymptomatic but have unexplained elevations in inflammatory markers, GCA should be considered.

Treatment of Polymyalgia Rheumatica

Glucocorticoids
Glucocorticoids are the cornerstone of treatment of PMR. The treatment duration for PMR varies among patients, with a mean duration of around 20 months.[43] The recommended initial prednisone dose ranges between 12.5 and 25 mg/d. This dose could be tapered to 10 mg daily by 4 to 8 weeks if tolerated, then by 1 mg every 2 to 4 weeks thereafter. For relapses, the dose should be increased to the prerelapse dose then tapered more gradually.

Steroid-sparing agents
When compared with GCA, patients with PMR require smaller doses of glucocorticoids. The risk versus benefit of adding a steroid-sparing agent should be weighed against the risk of low-dose prednisone.

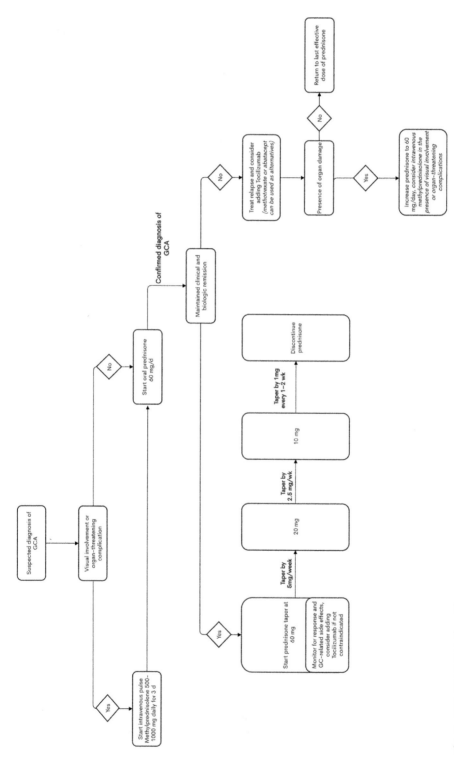

Fig. 2. GCA treatment algorithm.

Previous trials have shown mixed results with MTX treatment in PMR. All of them were small studies and used doses of MTX equal to or less than 10 mg/wk.[44–48] The first trial published in 1996 showed no steroid-sparing effect with the use of 7.5 mg weekly MTX.[46] Other trials showed a decrease in the cumulative dose of prednisone, duration of steroid treatment, and number of flare-ups in MTX groups.[45,47,48] There was no evidence that methotrexate decreased steroid-related side effects, although the studies were not powered adequately to detect that difference.[45,47] The authors recommend considering the use of methotrexate early on in patients at high risk of glucocorticoid-related side effect or in those with relapsing disease.

Limited data suggest that tocilizumab can be effective for isolated PMR[49] or in those with overlapping GCA.[30] TNF-inhibitors have not been found to be effective (**Fig. 2**).

CLINICS CARE POINTS

- GCA and PMR are most common in individuals of northern European descent who are 50 years or older.
- At the time of confirmed diagnosis of GCA, screening for large vessel involvement should be completed with noninvasive imaging modalities. Follow-up imaging is recommended in cases of known large vessel complications, inability to taper glucocorticoids or persistently elevated inflammatory markers.
- The addition of tocilizumab to glucocorticoids has been demonstrated to be effective at preventing relapses and shortening the duration of glucocorticoid therapy in 2 large randomized controlled trials.
- The diagnosis of PMR is based on consistent clinical symptoms, including proximal muscle pain and stiffness in the hip and shoulder girdle regions, a rapid response to moderate-dose prednisone (15–25 mg daily) and exclusion of common mimics.
- Glucocorticoid monotherapy is the cornerstone of treatment in PMR, with doses greater than 25 mg daily of prednisone rarely needed.

DISCLOSURE

The authors have nothing to disclose that is relevant to this article.

REFERENCES

1. Gonzalez-Gay MA, Vazquez-Rodriguez TR, Lopez-Diaz MJ, et al. Epidemiology of giant cell arteritis and polymyalgia rheumatica. Arthritis Rheum 2009;61(10): 1454–61.
2. de Boysson H, Liozon E, Ly KH, et al. The different clinical patterns of giant cell arteritis. Clin Exp Rheumatol 2019;37:57–60. Suppl 117 (2).
3. Hernandez-Rodriguez J, Murgia G, Villar I, et al. Description and Validation of Histological Patterns and Proposal of a Dynamic Model of Inflammatory Infiltration in Giant-cell Arteritis. Medicine (Baltimore) 2016;95(8):e2368.
4. Lie JT, Brown AL Jr, Carter ET. Spectrum of aging changes in temporal arteries. Its significance, in interpretation of biopsy of temporal artery. Arch Pathol 1970; 90(3):278–85.
5. Bowling K, Rait J, Atkinson J, et al. Temporal artery biopsy in the diagnosis of giant cell arteritis: Does the end justify the means? Ann Med Surg (Lond) 2017; 20:1–5.

6. Mahr A, Saba M, Kambouchner M, et al. Temporal artery biopsy for diagnosing giant cell arteritis: the longer, the better? Ann Rheum Dis 2006;65(6):826–8.

7. Durling B, Toren A, Patel V, et al. Incidence of discordant temporal artery biopsy in the diagnosis of giant cell arteritis. Can J Ophthalmol 2014;49(2):157–61.

8. Achkar AA, Lie JT, Hunder GG, et al. How does previous corticosteroid treatment affect the biopsy findings in giant cell (temporal) arteritis? Ann Intern Med 1994; 120(12):987–92.

9. Bley TA, Uhl M, Carew J, et al. Diagnostic value of high-resolution MR imaging in giant cell arteritis. AJNR Am J Neuroradiol 2007;28(9):1722–7.

10. Ghinoi A, Zuccoli G, Nicolini A, et al. 1T magnetic resonance imaging in the diagnosis of giant cell arteritis: comparison with ultrasonography and physical examination of temporal arteries. Clin Exp Rheumatol 2008;26(3 Suppl 49):S76–80.

11. Bley TA, Weiben O, Uhl M, et al. Assessment of the cranial involvement pattern of giant cell arteritis with 3T magnetic resonance imaging. Arthritis Rheum 2005; 52(8):2470–7.

12. Klink T, Geiger J, Both M, et al. Giant cell arteritis: diagnostic accuracy of MR imaging of superficial cranial arteries in initial diagnosis-results from a multicenter trial. Radiology 2014;273(3):844–52.

13. Luqmani R, Lee E, Singh S, et al. The Role of Ultrasound Compared to Biopsy of Temporal Arteries in the Diagnosis and Treatment of Giant Cell Arteritis (TABUL): a diagnostic accuracy and cost-effectiveness study. Health Technol Assess 2016;20(90):1–238.

14. Bley TA, Reinhard M, Hauenstein C, et al. Comparison of duplex sonography and high-resolution magnetic resonance imaging in the diagnosis of giant cell (temporal) arteritis. Arthritis Rheum 2008;58(8):2574–8.

15. Nuenninghoff DM, Hunder GG, Christianson TJ, et al. Mortality of large-artery complication (aortic aneurysm, aortic dissection, and/or large-artery stenosis) in patients with giant cell arteritis: a population-based study over 50 years. Arthritis Rheum 2003;48(12):3532–7.

16. Grayson PC, Tomasson G, Cuthbertson D, et al. Association of vascular physical examination findings and arteriographic lesions in large vessel vasculitis. J Rheumatol 2012;39(2):303–9.

17. de Boysson H, Aouba A. [The additional value of imaging (excluding Doppler) for the diagnosis and follow-up of giant cell arteritis]. Presse Med 2019;48(9): 931–40.

18. Loffler C, Hoffend J, Benck U, et al. The value of ultrasound in diagnosing extracranial large-vessel vasculitis compared to FDG-PET/CT: A retrospective study. Clin Rheumatol 2017;36(9):2079–86.

19. Hauenstein C, Reinhard M, Geiger J, et al. Effects of early corticosteroid treatment on magnetic resonance imaging and ultrasonography findings in giant cell arteritis. Rheumatology (Oxford) 2012;51(11):1999–2003.

20. Kermani TA, Schmidt J, Crowson CS, et al. Utility of erythrocyte sedimentation rate and C-reactive protein for the diagnosis of giant cell arteritis. Semin Arthritis Rheum 2012;41(6):866–71.

21. Mazlumzadeh M, Hunder GG, Easley KA, et al. Treatment of giant cell arteritis using induction therapy with high-dose glucocorticoids: a double-blind, placebo-controlled, randomized prospective clinical trial. Arthritis Rheum 2006;54(10): 3310–8.

22. Chevalet P, Barrier JH, Pottier P, et al. A randomized, multicenter, controlled trial using intravenous pulses of methylprednisolone in the initial treatment of simple

forms of giant cell arteritis: a one year followup study of 164 patients. J Rheumatol 2000;27(6):1484–91.

23. Hellmich B, Agueda A, Monti S, et al. 2018 Update of the EULAR recommendations for the management of large vessel vasculitis. Ann Rheum Dis 2020;79(1): 19–30.

24. Mackie SL, Dejaco C, Appenzeller S, et al. British Society for Rheumatology guideline on diagnosis and treatment of giant cell arteritis. Rheumatology (Oxford) 2020;59(3):e1–23.

25. Behn AR, Perera T, Myles AB. Polymyalgia rheumatica and corticosteroids: how much for how long? Ann Rheum Dis 1983;42(4):374–8.

26. Hachulla E, Boivin V, Pasturel-Michon U, et al. Prognostic factors and long-term evolution in a cohort of 133 patients with giant cell arteritis. Clin Exp Rheumatol 2001;19(2):171–6.

27. Hunder GG, Sheps SG, Allen GL, et al. Daily and alternate-day corticosteroid regimens in treatment of giant cell arteritis: comparison in a prospective study. Ann Intern Med 1975;82(5):613–8.

28. Villiger PM, Adler S, Kuchen S, et al. Tocilizumab for induction and maintenance of remission in giant cell arteritis: a phase 2, randomised, double-blind, placebo-controlled trial. Lancet 2016;387(10031):1921–7.

29. Xie F, Yun H, Bernatsky S, et al. Brief Report: Risk of Gastrointestinal Perforation Among Rheumatoid Arthritis Patients Receiving Tofacitinib, Tocilizumab, or Other Biologic Treatments. Arthritis Rheumatol 2016;68(11):2612–7.

30. Stone JH, Tuckwell K, Dimonaco S, et al. Trial of Tocilizumab in Giant-Cell Arteritis. N Engl J Med 2017;377(4):317–28.

31. Unizony S, Arias-Urdaneta L, Miloslavsky E, et al. Tocilizumab for the treatment of large-vessel vasculitis (giant cell arteritis, Takayasu arteritis) and polymyalgia rheumatica. Arthritis Care Res (Hoboken) 2012;64(11):1720–9.

32. Stone JH, Bao M, Han J, et al. Long-Term Outcome of Tocilizumab for Patients with Giant Cell Arteritis: Results from Part 2 of the Giacta Trial. Ann Rheum Dis 2019;78:145–6.

33. Nishimoto N, Miyasaka N, Yamamoto K, et al. Long-term safety and efficacy of tocilizumab, an anti-IL-6 receptor monoclonal antibody, in monotherapy, in patients with rheumatoid arthritis (the STREAM study): evidence of safety and efficacy in a 5-year extension study. Ann Rheum Dis 2009;68(10):1580–4.

34. Spiera RF, Mitnick HJ, Kupersmith M, et al. A prospective, double-blind, randomized, placebo controlled trial of methotrexate in the treatment of giant cell arteritis (GCA). Clin Exp Rheumatol 2001;19(5):495–501.

35. Jover JA, Hernandez-Garcia C, Morado IC, et al. Combined treatment of giant-cell arteritis with methotrexate and prednisone. a randomized, double-blind, placebo-controlled trial. Ann Intern Med 2001;134(2):106–14.

36. Hoffman GS, Cid MC, Hellmann DB, et al. A multicenter, randomized, double-blind, placebo-controlled trial of adjuvant methotrexate treatment for giant cell arteritis. Arthritis Rheum 2002;46(5):1309–18.

37. Mahr AD, Jover JA, Spiera RF, et al. Adjunctive methotrexate for treatment of giant cell arteritis: an individual patient data meta-analysis. Arthritis Rheum 2007; 56(8):2789–97.

38. Salvarani C, Della Bella C, Cimino L, et al. Risk factors for severe cranial ischaemic events in an Italian population-based cohort of patients with giant cell arteritis. Rheumatology (Oxford) 2009;48(3):250–3.

39. Nesher G, Berkun Y, Mates M, et al. Low-dose aspirin and prevention of cranial ischemic complications in giant cell arteritis. Arthritis Rheum 2004;50(4):1332–7.

40. Narvaez J, Bernad B, Nolla JM, et al. Statin therapy does not seem to benefit giant cell arteritis. Semin Arthritis Rheum 2007;36(5):322–7.

41. Salvarani C, Cantini F, Hunder GG. Polymyalgia rheumatica and giant-cell arteritis. Lancet 2008;372(9634):234–45.

42. Raheel S, Shbeeb I, Crowson CS, et al. Epidemiology of Polymyalgia Rheumatica 2000-2014 and Examination of Incidence and Survival Trends Over 45 Years: A Population-Based Study. Arthritis Care Res (Hoboken) 2017;69(8):1282–5.

43. Chuang TY, Hunder GG, Ilstrup DM, et al. Polymyalgia rheumatica: a 10-year epidemiologic and clinical study. Ann Intern Med 1982;97(5):672–80.

44. van der Veen MJ, Dinant HJ, van Booma-Frankfort C, et al. Can methotrexate be used as a steroid sparing agent in the treatment of polymyalgia rheumatica and giant cell arteritis? Ann Rheum Dis 1996;55(4):218–23.

45. Ferraccioli G, Salaffi F, De Vita S, et al. Methotrexate in polymyalgia rheumatica: preliminary results of an open, randomized study. J Rheumatol 1996;23(4):624–8.

46. Feinberg HL, Sherman JD, Schrepferman CG, et al. The use of methotrexate in polymyalgia rheumatica. J Rheumatol 1996;23(9):1550–2.

47. Cimmino MA, Salvarani C, Macchioni P, et al. Long-term follow-up of polymyalgia rheumatica patients treated with methotrexate and steroids. Clin Exp Rheumatol 2008;26(3):395–400.

48. Caporali R, Cimmino MA, Ferraccioli G, et al. Prednisone plus methotrexate for polymyalgia rheumatica: a randomized, double-blind, placebo-controlled trial. Ann Intern Med 2004;141(7):493–500.

49. Macchioni P, Boiardi L, Catanoso M, et al. Tocilizumab for polymyalgia rheumatica: report of two cases and review of the literature. Semin Arthritis Rheum 2013;43(1):113–8.

Suspecting and Diagnosing the Patient with Spondyloarthritis and What to Expect from Therapy

Philip J. Mease, MD, MACR[a,b,*]

KEYWORDS

- Spondyloarthritis • Axial spondyloarthritis • Psoriatic arthritis • Reactive arthritis
- Inflammatory bowel disease arthritis • Ankylosing spondylitis

KEY POINTS

- Understanding of the clinical presentation, natural history, epidemiology, and pathogenesis of the spondyloarthritides is rapidly evolving. The disease is more common than previously recognized.
- Because of the array of clinical manifestations, it may be difficult to recognize the spondyloarthritides in their various clinical manifestations.
- Case finding and appropriate referral to a rheumatologist are important to treat spondylarthritis early for the best opportunity to achieve remission or low disease activity.
- Advances in treatment of the spondyloarthritides have been dramatic, allowing us to potentially achieve remission or low disease activity for most patients.

INTRODUCTION

Although the spondyloarthritides have been recognized in the medical literature for more than 100 years, the understanding of their distinct genetics, pathophysiology, and clinical presentation is still in evolution, as is a true understanding of their epidemiology. Although spondyloarthritis (SpA) (preferred term over "spondyloarthropathy") is optimally considered a singular overarching disease concept, clinicians who initially recognize and those who confirm diagnosis and manage these patients have historically balkanized SpA into several subsets: ankylosing spondylitis (AS), psoriatic

This article originally appeared in the Medical Clinics of North America, Volume 105, Issue 2, March 2021.
[a] Rheumatology Research, Swedish Medical Center/Providence St. Joseph Health, Seattle, WA, USA; [b] University of Washington School of Medicine, Seattle, WA, USA
* 601 Broadway, Suite 600, Seattle, WA 98122.
E-mail address: pmease@philipmease.com

Rheum Dis Clin N Am 48 (2022) 507–521
https://doi.org/10.1016/j.rdc.2022.02.008
0889-857X/22/© 2022 Elsevier Inc. All rights reserved.

arthritis (PsA), the arthritis associated with inflammatory bowel disease (IBD), reactive arthritis (ReA; associated with a triggering infection), and undifferentiated SpA, the last for placing those who clinically behave like SpA but do not fall into one of the other subsets. The 7 blind men and the elephant metaphor can be applied here. For example, a spine orthopedist or physiatrist, when encountering a young male patient with persistent back pain and prominent morning stiffness, out of proportion to radiographic findings, may consider the diagnosis of AS. A dermatologist who is treating a patient with psoriasis, upon encountering a dactylitic finger (complete swelling of a digit), considers PsA. An internist whose patient has developed polyarticular tenderness and swelling as well as disabling pain at the Achilles tendon insertion (a manifestation of enthesitis) after having a bout of diarrhea while traveling in Central America considers the condition ReA (historically known as "Reiter syndrome"). An ophthalmologist, seeing a young patient with acute anterior uveitis, asks the patient if they have had back pain or arthritis, considering some form of SpA. A gastroenterologist reading an MRI enterography report on a patient with Crohn disease, in which the radiologist comments that the patient "lights up" not only in the intestine but also in the sacroiliac (SI) joints, considers the form of SpA that accompanies IBD. In all of these instances, it is hoped, these considerations will prompt referral of the patient to a rheumatologist to help sort out whether a SpA is present, distinguishing it from other musculoskeletal and inflammatory diseases, such as degenerative arthritis of the spine or peripheral joints, rheumatoid arthritis (RA), gout, fibromyalgia (FM), or other disorders. Part of the "sorting" is the recognition that the diagnosis may not be "either-or"; it is very common to have more than one of these conditions simultaneously, especially as degenerative joint disease occurs in virtually every human as we age. The key point of a rheumatologic consultation will be to sort whether an immunologic inflammatory disease is present, because we now have an evolving pharmacopeia of advanced therapies, including immunologically targeted biologic and synthetic disease-modifying drugs (DMARDs) with which we are potentially able to achieve disease remission or low disease activity.

SPONDYLOARTHRITIS BACKGROUND AND HISTORY

It may come as a surprise to the reader that the prevalence of all forms of SpA is up to 2% of the general population in most parts of the world, with some geographic differences based on population genetic differences. RA occurs in approximately 1% of the general population, yet tends to be more recognized by clinicians and the public. Part of the reason for lack of recognition of the spondyloarthritides is the historical subsetting of SpA into different disease entities that are not as well understood or recognized, leading to frequent misdiagnosis or lack of diagnosis. The SpA conditions have been noted in the archeologic record dating at least back to the fifth century AD, with skeletal osseous changes consistent with PsA recovered from ruins of Christian monasteries where people with psoriasis (considered to be leprosy) sheltered, and even before, in Egyptian mummies with spinal osseous changes consistent either with SpA or diffuse idiopathic skeletal hyperostosis. Nevertheless, the classification of SpA was not codified until the 1961 Rome criteria for AS. In the mid-1970s, Moll and colleagues[1] distinguished the SpA conditions from RA as typically seronegative for rheumatoid factor antibody and variably manifest with spinal involvement, asymmetric peripheral arthritis, enthesitis (inflammation of tendon and ligament attachments to bone), and association with IBD, psoriasis, and uveitis. It was during this same period that association with the gene marker HLA-B27 was noted,[2] and Calin and colleagues[3] developed the first criteria set for "inflammatory back pain" (IBP) to help clinicians distinguish it, through patient history, from degenerative or mechanical back pain. In 1984, the modified New York (mNY) criteria for the classification of AS was published, which anchored the disease in radiographically visible SI joint damage along with several clinical features.[4] Since that time, especially with the introduction of advanced imaging technology such as MRI, wider application of genetic testing, and increased awareness of a broader spectrum of clinical presentation representing SpA, various updated classification criteria have been put forward.[5,6] In 2006, the CASPAR criteria for the classification of PsA was published, based on a study of nearly 1000 patients with either PsA or another inflammatory arthritis condition, yielding a specificity of 99% and sensitivity of 93%[7] (**Box 1**).

Axial Spondyloarthritis Classification Criteria

The reader is referred to a current review of the general topic of axial spondyloarthritis (AxSpA), which has been recently published as a textbook.[8] In 2009, the Assessment of SpondyloArthritis International Society (ASAS) group published classification criteria for AxSpA,[9] and in 2011, for peripheral spondyloarthritis (pSpA)[10] (**Figs. 1 and 2**). The ASAS criteria reflect a more clinically practical recognition that patients with SpA tend to present with either predominantly axial manifestations or predominantly peripheral features, including peripheral arthritis, enthesitis, and dactylitis, albeit acknowledging that overlap can occur. Patients with AxSpA may either have classic radiographic changes in the SI joints (eg, periarticular sclerosis, joint space narrowing, erosions, ankylosis) or MRI changes consistent with inflammation of the

---

Box 1
The CASPAR criteria

To meet the CASPAR (ClASsification criteria for Psoriatic ARthritis) criteria, a patient must have inflammatory articular disease (joint, spine, or entheseal) with ≥3 points from the following 5 categories:

1. Evidence of current psoriasis, a personal history of psoriasis, or a family history of psoriasis.
   Current psoriasis is defined as psoriatic skin or scalp disease present today as judged by a rheumatologist or dermatologist.[a]
   A personal history of psoriasis is defined as a history of psoriasis that may be obtained from a patient, family physician, dermatologist, rheumatologist, or other qualified health care provider.
   A family history of psoriasis is defined as a history of psoriasis in a first- or second-degree relative according to patient report.
2. Typical psoriatic nail dystrophy, including onycholysis, pitting, and hyperkeratosis, observed on current physical examination.
3. A negative test result for the presence of rheumatoid factor by any method except latex but preferably by enzyme-linked immunosorbent assay or nephelometry, according to the local laboratory reference range.
4. Either current dactylitis, defined as swelling of an entire digit, or a history of dactylitis recorded by a rheumatologist.
5. Radiographic evidence of juxtaarticular new bone formation, appearing as ill-defined ossification near joint margins (but excluding osteophyte formation) on plain radiographs of the hand or foot.

The CASPAR criteria have specificity of 98.7% and sensitivity of 91.4%.[a] Current psoriasis is assigned a score of 2; all other features are assigned a score of 1.

From Taylor W, Gladman D, Helliwell P, et al. Classification criteria for psoriatic arthritis: development of new criteria from a large international study. Arthritis Rheum 2006;54(8):2671; with permission.

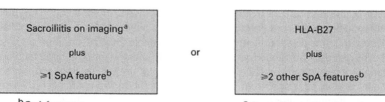

b SpA features:
- Inflammatory back pain
- Arthritis
- Enthesitis (heel)
- Uveitis
- Dactylitis
- Psoriasis
- Crohn's disease/ulcerative colitis
- Good response to NSAIDs
- Family history for SpA
- HLA-B27
- Elevated CRP

a Sacroiliitis on imaging:
- Active (acute) inflammation on MRI highly suggestive of sacroiliitis associated with SpA
  or
- Definite radiographic sacroiliitis according to mod. New York criteria

Fig. 1. ASAS classification criteria for AxSpA (in patients with back pain > 3 months and age at onset < 45 years). Sensitivity 82.9%, specificity 84.4%; n = 649 patients with chronic back pain and age at onset < 45 years. Imaging arm (sacroiliitis) alone has a sensitivity of 66.2% and a specificity of 97.3%. **Note: Elevated CRP is considered a SpA feature in the context of chronic back pain. (*From* Rudwaleit M, Landewé R, van der Heijde D, et al. The development of Assessment of SpondyloArthritis international Society classification criteria for axial spondyloarthritis (part II): validation and final selection. Ann Rheum Dis 2009;68(6):777-83; with permission.)

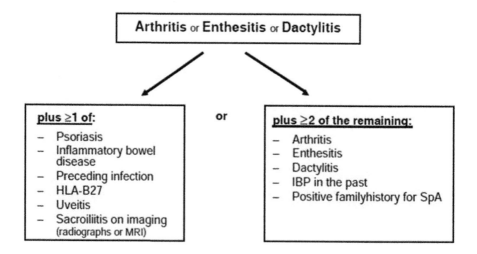

Sensitivity: 77.8%; Specificity: 82.2%

Fig. 2. ASAS classification criteria for peripheral SpA. (*Adapted from* Rudwaleit M, van der Heijde D, Landewé R, et al. The Assessment of SpondyloArthritis International Society classification criteria for peripheral spondyloarthritis and for spondyloarthritis in general. Ann Rheum Dis 2011;70(1):28; with permission.)

Box 2
Inflammatory back pain (Assessment of SpondyloArthritis International Society criteria)

1. Age at onset less than 40 years

2. Insidious onset

3. Improvement with exercise

4. No improvement with rest

5. Pain at night (with improvement upon getting up)

IBP if 4/5 are present.

Sensitivity 79.6%; specificity 72.4%.

From Sieper J, van der Heijde D, Landewé R, et al. New criteria for inflammatory back pain in patients with chronic back pain: a real patient exercise by experts from the Assessment of SpondyloArthritis international Society (ASAS). Ann Rheum Dis 2009;68(6):784-8; with permission.

SI joints (periarticular bone edema) plus 1 other characteristic SpA feature, such as IBP (**Box 2**) or a positive HLA-B27 gene marker plus at least 2 characteristic SpA features. Those patients with characteristic radiographic changes of the SI joint are considered to be synonymous with those formerly classified by the mNY criteria with AS, and those without these radiographic features are, for the moment, being called "nonradiographic" axial spondyloarthritis. The term "axial spondyloarthritis" reflects the larger set of patients now included, many of whom do not have classic ankylosis of the spine or SI joints. Population studies in the United States suggest that AS, or radiographic AxSpA, is present in 0.5% of the population, whereas the broader set of patients may be present in up to 1.4% of the population. Whereas AS is considered to be present in a 2:1 male-to-female proportion, the full spectrum of AxSpA is considered to be equi-gender, an important point for the clinician to consider when evaluating a woman with back pain. Whereas some patients may present with radiographic and/or MRI changes in the spine consistent with AxSpA, there can be many "false positive" changes in the spine, thus the focus in these criteria on changes in the SI joints, which are less likely to show false positive changes than the spine. It is important to take in the "stem" of the criteria, that is, that in order to apply the criteria, the symptoms of the condition should be chronic, and onset should be before the age of 45.

Peripheral Spondyloarthritis Classification Criteria

The pSpA criteria include peripheral arthritis (typically asymmetric and predominantly lower limb), enthesitis, or dactylitis plus either one or 2 characteristic SpA features[10] (see **Fig. 2**). Although, classically, SpA subsets, such as PsA, the arthritis of IBD, ReA, and undifferentiated SpA, present more peripherally and thus tend to be categorized in this set, there can be considerable overlap with AxSpA features[11] (**Fig. 3**). For example, axial involvement may occur in up to 40% of PsA patients, such that such a patient may be simultaneously classifiable as having PsA and AxSpA (either radiographic or nonradiographic). Intriguingly, the axial manifestations seen in PsA may differ from classic AxSpA in that spine involvement may appear at an older age, sacroiliitis may be unilateral, spinal syndesmophytes may have a different morphologic appearance, there may be more cervical spine involvement, and there may be different genetic markers, for example, HLA-B8 positivity. Furthermore, it has been shown that the CASPAR criteria, developed specifically for PsA classification, are

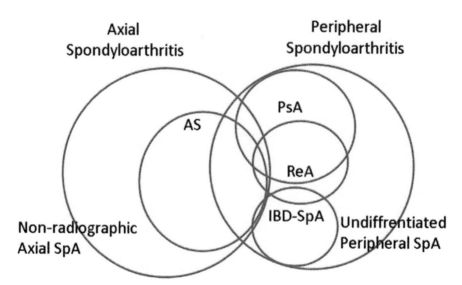

Fig. 3. Spectrum of SpA: current concept. (*From* Raychaudhuri SP, Deodhar A. The classification and diagnostic criteria of ankylosing spondylitis. J Autoimmun 2014;48-49:129; with permission.)

more reliable in positively identifying true positive cases and excluding negative ones compared with the ASAS pSpA criteria.[10] In ReA, the spinal involvement may be more transient than is classic for AxSpA. It is recognized that as the understanding of SpA continues to mature, there will likely be further evolution of the classification criteria, which in the future will likely include genotype and other disease-specific serum biomarkers that will allow more precise categorization of patients for diagnostic and treatment stratification purposes.

In the previous historical survey of the SpA concept, note the emphasis on classification criteria. Such criteria are useful particularly for research purposes, when one is trying to identify a more homogeneous group to study disease characteristics, comorbidity frequency, and effects of treatment. Thus, such criteria ideally should have a high specificity, which may be at the expense of sensitivity, meaning that some true positive cases may not be included, for example, patients that have disease onset after the age of 45 in the case of AxSpA. In order for the classification criteria to be applied to a patient, one should first have clinical diagnostic judgment that the patient could possibly have an SpA condition.In particular, being aware of a possible SpA condition may be a challenge for nonrheumatologists as they try to distinguish if an immunologic, inflammatory condition could be accounting for at least a portion, if not all, of a patient's symptoms of back pain, peripheral arthritis, enthesitis, and other features. Although there are no formal diagnostic criteria for the spondyloarthritides, if enough characteristic features identified through history, family history, physical examination, laboratory testing, and imaging are present, then the patient is certainly appropriate for referral to a rheumatologist, and then, depending on the rheumatologist's judgment about diagnosis and disease severity, worthy of progressing up the treatment ladder. Sometimes even expert rheumatologists cannot be certain, and a diagnosis becomes more certain, positive or negative, after seeing the results of treatment trials. Just as much care needs to be taken to not overdiagnose to avoid treatment that may be expensive or harmful, as to underdiagnose and miss the opportunity to effectively treat disease. The following sections provide approaches to effective differential diagnosis of SpA, beginning with AxSpA and progressing to other forms of SpA.

Axial Spondyloarthritis Diagnosis

A key starting point in sorting out AxSpA is to ask 5 key IBP criteria questions[12] (see **Box 2**). Did the pain that is characteristic of the patient's back pain begin before the age of 40? Did the pain problem gradually grow on them (insidious) rather than being sudden in onset? Does pain get better as the patient moves about and is active? Is there no improvement in pain with rest? Does the pain awaken the patient at night, especially in the second half of the night, and improves if the patient gets up? If the answer is "yes" to at least 4 of these 5 questions, then the possibility of an inflammatory condition is increased. A corollary question is are they particularly stiff when first moving about, and how long does it take for stiffness to resolve; is it sometimes more than an hour? As can be seen in **Fig. 4**, the responses to these questions will likely be different if the main reason for the back pain is degenerative/mechanical or a problem such as an infection or malignancy. Rudwaleit and colleagues[13] have identified additional features in addition to IBP that cumulatively increase the likelihood that the 5% of chronic back pain patients who have IBP may ultimately have a diagnosis of AxSpA (**Table 1**). Additional features include accompanying peripheral arthritis, typically asymmetric and lower extremity, persistent pain around the heel (Achilles or plantar fascia enthesitis), dactylitis (sausage digit), family history of an SpA condition, a good response to nonsteroidal anti-inflammatory drugs (NSAIDs), a history of an

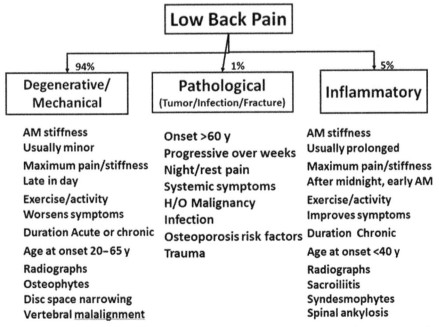

Fig. 4. Low back pain. (*From* Sieper J, van der Heijde D, Landewé R, et al. New criteria for inflammatory back pain in patients with chronic back pain: a real patient exercise by experts from the Assessment of SpondyloArthritis international Society (ASAS). Ann Rheum Dis 2009;68(6):784-8; with permission.). H/O, History of.

Table 1
Clinical utility of the clinical parameters of SpA

	Sensitivity	Specificity	+LR
Inflammatory back pain (updated information)	80%	72%	2.9
Enthesitis (heel pain)	37%	89%	3.4
Peripheral arthritis	40	90	4.0
Dactylitis	18	96	4.5
Acute anterior uveitis	22	97	7.3
Positive family history for AS, AAU, IBD, ReA	32	95	6.4
Psoriasis	10	96	2.5
Inflammatory bowel disease	4	99	4.0
Good response to NSAIDs	77	85	5.1
↑ acute phase reactants	50	80	2.5
HLA-B27 *(updated information)*	*Variable*	*Variable*	11
MRI (STIR) sacroiliitis *(updated information)*	*Variable*	*Variable*	11

Abbreviation: LR, Likelihood ratio; SIJ, sacroiliac joints.
 Adapted from Rudwaleit M, van der Heijde D, Khan MA, et al. How to diagnose axial spondyloar-thritis early. Ann Rheum Dis 2004;63(5):535-43; with permission.

associated condition, such as psoriasis, IBD, or uveitis, and objective laboratory testing and imaging, such as a positive HLA-B27 test, elevated C-reactive protein (CRP), or MRI findings characteristic of SpA. An algorithmic approach to diagnosis has been suggested by van den Berg and colleagues[14] (**Fig. 5**) in which a patient with the proper "stem," that is, has chronic back pain with onset less than 45 years

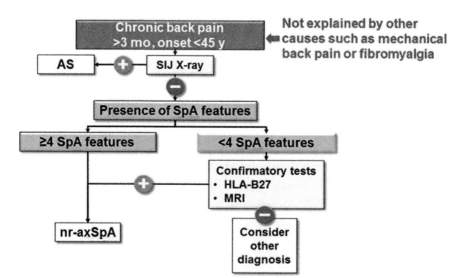

Fig. 5. How should we diagnose axial SpA in practice? (*From* van den Berg R, de Hooge M, Rudwaleit M, et al. ASAS modification of the Berlin algorithm for diagnosing axial spondyloarthritis: results from the SPondyloArthritis Caught Early (SPACE)-cohort and from the Assessment of SpondyloArthritis international Society (ASAS)-cohort. Ann Rheum Dis 2013;72(10):1646-53; with permission.)

of age, has either a pelvis radiograph consistent with sacroiliitis, leading to a diagnosis of AS, or has a normal SI radiograph, but does have other characteristic SpA features, prompting further evaluation. If enough of these features are present, triage to a rheumatologist is appropriate.

Take note of the focus on radiographic evaluation of SI joints; a plain pelvis radiograph will do. It is all too common for a patient to have multiple sets of lumbar spine radiographs and MRI scans that show modest degenerative changes, yet no attention to the SI joints. There has been controversy about how to best radiographically image the SI joints, partly because the local radiologist may have been taught that angled views of the joints are best because the joint runs at an angle to the anteroposterior (AP) plane. However, there is risk of increased radiation exposure as the radiology technician makes several attempts to get the correct angled shot. The SpA research community's most common recommendation is that a single AP view will suffice. Regardless of radiographic technique, numerous studies have shown that there is significant variation in what is considered truly abnormal, and to what degree, especially with intermediate grades of abnormality. MRI is more sensitive and reliable to give information about the presence of inflammation as well as damage. Computed tomography (CT) scan can provide exquisite detail about damage, albeit at the expense of radiation exposure. For this reason, low-dose CT is now beginning to be used. Beyond radiograph, it is probably best to leave ordering of advanced imaging up to the rheumatologist, who may have a special understanding about technique with local musculoskeletal radiologists.

The only laboratory studies for AxSpA are the CRP—we rely on this more so than erythrocyte sedimentation rate (ESR)—and the HLA-B27 gene marker. Other autoimmune disease–related autoantibodies or disease activity markers may be assessed, for example, to rule out RA, lupus, and so forth, in the differential diagnosis, but are not used to rule in SpA. Note that the CRP is often not elevated in SpA, even with active disease, so if normal, it is not necessarily helpful, unless it has become normal with effective treatment. Similarly, HLA-B27 may be negative in up to 20% of classic AS and even more in other subtypes. Furthermore, HLA-B27 varies with race, for example, being present less frequently in African Americans but more frequently in certain Native American populations. Thus, one cannot rely on any laboratory testing for reliable diagnostic purposes. Discovery of biomarkers that can more reliably be used for diagnosis or evaluating disease severity remains an unmet need and is an active area of research.

Peripheral Spondyloarthritis Diagnosis

In a similar way, diagnosis and monitoring of patients with primarily peripheral, or mixed peripheral and axial SpA, are a matter of pattern recognition of symptoms, such as persistent pain arising from inflammation in joints, sites of tendon and ligament insertion into bone (classically around the heel, knee, pelvis, thorax, shoulder, and elbow), and swelling of a whole digit, known as dactylitis. The presence of a genetically associated condition, such as IBD, psoriasis, and uveitis, or a family history of the same or similar autoimmune disease is an important clue for diagnosis. The most common form of SpA presenting in this manner is PsA. Psoriasis occurs in 3.2% of the US population.[15] PsA occurs in up to 30% of patients with psoriasis in North America and Western Europe.[16] In most patients, psoriasis precedes the onset of PsA, by, on average, 10 years, but in some, the skin manifestations develop at the same time as musculoskeletal symptoms, whereas, in a few, the skin manifestations follow the appearance of arthritic and entheseal ones. Because of the first appearance of skin and nail disease, clinicians caring for these manifestations, for example, dermatologists and primary care physicians, are in the best position to be monitoring patients for musculoskeletal symptoms suggestive of PsA in order to triage the patient to rheumatologists for early treatment. Certain patient-reported questionnaires, such as the PEST[17] can help with case finding by questioning if there has been any history of joint swelling, a diagnosis of arthritis, nail pitting, pain in the heel (enthesitis), or swelling of a whole digit (dactylitis). In the early stages of PsA, oligoarticular involvement (<5 inflamed joints) is common, but as the disease matures, polyarticular presentation is the norm. Distal interphalangeal (DIP) joints are frequently involved, unlike RA, and may make it difficult to discern from osteoarthritis changes of DIP joints. Enthesitis is present in 30% to 70%, dactylitis in 40% to 50%, and spine disease in up to 50% of PsA patients.[18] Spine disease includes sacroiliitis, often asymmetric, nonmarginal syndesmophytes, and frequent cervical spine involvement, features that distinguish axial PsA from classic AxSpA.[19,20] Radiographs and advanced imaging, such as ultrasound (US) and MRI, are diagnostically useful, and US and MRI can distinguish inflammatory arthritis and enthesitis from degenerative disease and FM. As in AxSpA, there is a paucity of laboratory biomarkers to diagnose PsA. CRP is elevated in less than half the patients, even with active disease. HLA-B27 may be present in patients with axial presentation. Although rheumatoid factor and cyclic citrullinated peptide are typically negative, in a small percentage of patients, they may be positive, so positivity of these tests cannot rule out PsA.

Inflammatory bowel disease

Musculoskeletal symptoms, including oligoarticular arthritis, polyarthritis, polyarthralgias, and spondylitis, occur in 10% to 20% of patients with IBD, more so with Crohn than with ulcerative colitis. Associated conditions include uveitis, episcleritis, erythema nodosum, pyoderma gangrenosum, and psoriasis. The obvious clue to the cause of these symptoms is the presence of IBD.[21] As in PsA, the gastroenterology clinical staff should be sensitive to this association to improve case findings and prompt referral to rheumatology for evaluation and collaborative decision making about therapeutic approach.

Reactive arthritis

ReA, which used to be called Reiter syndrome, occurs as a sequela of a triggering infection with microbes, such as Salmonella, Shigella, Yersinia, Campylobacter, and Chlamydia, among others.[22] Accurate figures on incidence and prevalence are hard to come by. It appears that between 0.5% and 2% of infected individuals may present with ReA, based partly on genetic factors, including HLA-B27. Clinical symptoms include typically asymmetric arthritis, predominantly lower extremity, spondylitis, enthesitis, and/or dactylitis and relatively recent, not necessarily active, history of infection. Associated conditions can include conjunctivitis, uveitis, urethritis, erythema nodosum, and keratoderma blennorrhagica, the presence of which can help with the differential diagnosis. The natural history of most cases of ReA is to remit over the course of 3 months to 6 months, but some may develop a chronic course.

There are several comorbidities that are present in a higher prevalence in the spondyloarthritides, depending on the spondyloarthritis subset, than in the general population. Some of these include metabolic syndrome (obesity, hyperlipidemia, and hypertension), cardiovascular disease, nonalcoholic steatotic hepatitis, depression, and FM, to name a few.[23,24] Some of these comorbidities are modifiable, and when addressed, can improve disease outcomes. For example, this has been shown with weight reduction programs. Comanagement of cardiovascular comorbidity is especially important for the patient's health care team. When FM, partially synonymous with central sensitization syndrome, is coexistent, as can be seen in 10% to 30% of patient cohorts, measures of disease activity that include subjective elements will typically be worse. When these measures are used as targets of treatment, patients with concomitant FM are less likely to achieve these targets. Concomitant FM needs to be recognized in order to avoid potentially unnecessary switching between immunomodulatory medicines, and efforts to treat FM should be instituted.[24]

Why does early identification of an SpA condition matter? Over the last 2 and a half decades, parallel advancements have been witnessed in both the understanding of the pathophysiology of SpA diseases and the development of increasingly effective treatment options that now allow routine achievement of remission or low disease activity, particularly in patients who do not have long delays in their diagnosis and treatment. A detailed review of pathophysiology is beyond the scope of this article; the reader is referred to several excellent reviews.[18,25–28] Although the balance of immune cell proliferation and activation and proinflammatory cytokine constituency will vary from 1 disease subset and 1 tissue domain (synovium, enthesium, bone, skin, gut, eye, and so forth) to another, there are certain commonalities between SpA subsets and their associated conditions. There appears to be a greater involvement of innate immune system activation than in more classically adaptive immune system diseases, such as RA. In other words, more "front-line" defense mechanisms at play responding to external-internal incitement, such as infections, perturbation in the gut or skin microbiome, mechanical microtrauma, and HLA-B27 unfolded protein response.[29] Dendritic and other cells then overproduce cytokines, such as interleukin-23 (IL-23), which migrates to potential sites of inflammation where both resident immune cells of the innate immune system and cells of the adaptive immune system are activated, producing more proinflammatory cytokines, including IL-17 and tumor necrosis factor-α (TNF-α). These cytokines, in turn, interact with receptors on effector cells, such as macrophages, neutrophils, other lymphocytes, keratinocytes, and osteoblasts, leading to inflammation and tissue destruction in synovium, bone, skin, and so forth. By targeting these proinflammatory cytokines and cells with specific inhibitors, inflammation and tissue destruction can be controlled, and in many cases, if treatment is maintained, the disease can be in a state of remission or near-remission.

TREATMENT

The landscape of treatment of the spondyloarthritides has undergone a revolutionary change in the last 2 decades because of the discovery and increasingly widespread use of medications that inhibit or regulate specific immunologic targets. Achieving outcomes, such as remission or low disease activity, are now reachable for our patients. The following is a brief review of the treatment "ladder" for the spondyloarthritides. It is within the purview of nonrheumatologists to initiate treatment of SpA patients with NSAIDs and nonnarcotic analgesics, as well as nonpharmacologic therapies, such as physical therapy. Glucocorticoids are avoided except to briefly treat flares. Traditionally, initiation of immunomodulatory medications has been left to the rheumatologist because of potential safety concerns with these agents and also because of the more recent proliferation of medications to choose from.[30–33] **Box 3**[34–36] and **Box 4**[37,38] include listings of various immunomodulatory medications and their classes that have shown efficacy in the treatment of SpA conditions, most of which have gained regulatory approval, although for some, approval is still pending. Fortunately, for patients, there has been an exponential growth of treatment options that can be effective. Efficacy is determined by assessing, through subjective questioning about symptoms, for example, pain and fatigue, physical examination, joint palpation for

---

Box 3
Psoriatic arthritis therapeutic groups

- Nonsteroidal anti-inflammatory drugs (NSAIDs)
- Conventional synthetic DMARDs (cs-DMARDs)
  - Methotrexate, sulfasalazine, leflunomide
- TNF inhibitors (TNFi)
  - Etanercept, infliximab, adalimumab, golimumab, certolizumab
- IL12/23i
  - Ustekinumab
- IL17i
  - Secukinumab, ixekizumab, brodalumab, bimekizumab
- IL23i
  - Guselkumab, risankizumab, tildrakizumab
- T-cell modulator
  - Abatacept
- Targeted synthetic DMARDs (ts-DMARDs)
  - PDE4i (apremilast)
  - JAKi (tofacitinib, baricitinib, upanacitinib, filgotinib)

Data from Mease PJ. Biologic Therapy for Psoriatic Arthritis. Rheum Dis Clin North Am 2015;41(4):723-38; and Mease PJ, Armstrong AW. Managing patients with psoriatic disease: the diagnosis and pharmacologic treatment of psoriatic arthritis in patients with psoriasis. Drugs 2014;74(4):423-41.

---

tenderness and swelling, entheseal insertion tenderness, finger swelling consistent with dactylitis, spine motion, and skin involvement. It is also assessed by measuring change in CRP, in those in whom CRP is elevated. One can also assess change in inflammation using US and MRI, and damage by radiograph. It is very common for a drug to work for a period of time and then lose adequate efficacy, so the optimal care of an SpA patient has to do with frequent quantification of disease severity (or absence thereof) and adjusting or switching medications to address changes.

Choice of therapy is individualized based on a shared decision-making process between patient and clinician. Does the patient have a preference for an oral option versus parenteral? For example, a frequent traveler may prefer an oral medicine because of ease of transport, or the person may be needle phobic. Are there cost implications of 1 choice over another? What clinical domains are most involved, and are

---

Box 4
Axial spondyloarthritis therapeutic groups

- Nonsteroidal anti-inflammatory drugs (NSAIDs)
- TNF inhibitors (TNFi)
  - Etanercept, infliximab, adalimumab, golimumab, certolizumab
- IL17i
  - Secukinumab, ixekizumab, bimekizumab
- Targeted synthetic DMARDs (ts-DMARDs)
  - JAKi (tofactinib, baricitinib, upanacitinib, filgotinib)

From Mease P. Emerging Immunomodulatory Therapies and New Treatment Paradigms for Axial Spondyloarthritis. Curr Rheumatol Rep 2019;21(7):35; with permission.

---

there specific safety concerns? If skin disease is severe, should an IL-17 inhibitor be chosen that yields better skin clearance? What if skin disease improves significantly but not the joints or vice versa; both outcomes can be seen unpredictably, necessitating course correction. If the patient has active uveitis and IBD along with musculoskeletal involvement, should a monoclonal antibody construct of TNF inhibitor be used that can benefit these manifestations as well as skin and musculoskeletal domains? Conversely, if IBD is present, should NSAIDs and IL-17 inhibitors be avoided? There is also the need for close monitoring of safety and tolerability of each medication. A common denominator concern with any immunomodulatory agent is the potential for increased infection. For some, there are also risks for malignancy (rare), allergic reactions, and laboratory abnormalities about which the patient needs to be educated and placed on a monitoring regimen. If the patient has frequent sinus infections with a therapy, should medicines be switched, seeking less frequent infection? If the patient develops a paradoxic TNF inhibitor-induced psoriasis or lupuslike syndrome, should the patient be switched to a different mechanism of action? In general, the benefit-cost ratio of disease control versus side effects comes down significantly on the side of benefit from disease control. Although for many patients, need for treatment is ongoing, in some, it is warranted to taper or stop medications if prolonged remission has been achieved. Treatment course is best determined through shared decision making between the patient and their care team. Ideally, members of the care team, for example, rheumatologists, primary care clinicians, dermatologists, gastroenterologists, ophthalmologists, physiatrists, orthopedists, and physical therapists, are communicating readily with each other.

CLINICS CARE POINTS

- Spondyloarthritis should be considered in patients presenting with chronic inflammatory back pain, peripheral arthritis, tendon or ligament insertion pain (enthesitis), especially if there are associated conditions, such as uveitis, IBD, or psoriasis.

- There are few laboratory abnormalities that can aid in diagnosis, other than CRP/ESR, which may be variably elevated, and the HLA B27 gene; thus, history and physical examination are critical in initial screening.

- Imaging, especially advanced imaging such as MRI of the pelvis and spine, to assess for inflammatory changes in bones and joints, or US of peripheral joints and entheses, can be helpful in diagnosis.

- Differential diagnosis with conditions such as osteoarthritis, degenerative spine disease, mechanical back pain or tendonitis, gout, and FM can be difficult to sort out. Referral to a rheumatologist is often warranted for the establishment of an accurate diagnosis.

- Once a diagnosis is made and effective therapy is initiated, coordinated teamwork between the rheumatologist, primary care physician, dermatologist, gastroenterologist, ophthalmologist, physiatrist, orthopedic surgeon, physical therapist, and other caregivers is optimal for patient management.

DISCLOSURE

Research grant, consultation fees, and/or speaker honoraria: AbbVie, Amgen, Boehringer Ingelheim, Bristol Myers Squibb, Eli Lilly, Galapagos, Gilead, GlaxoSmithKline, Janssen, Novartis, Pfizer, Sun, UCB.

REFERENCES

1. Moll JM, Haslock I, Macrae IF, et al. Associations between ankylosing spondylitis, psoriatic arthritis, Reiter's disease, the intestinal arthropathies, and Behcet's syndrome. Medicine (Baltimore) 1974;53(5):343–64.
2. Brewerton DA, Hart FD, Nicholls A, et al. Ankylosing spondylitis and HL-A 27. Lancet 1973;1(7809):904–7.
3. Calin A, Porta J, Fries JF, et al. Clinical history as a screening test for ankylosing spondylitis. JAMA 1977;237(24):2613–4.
4. van der Linden S, Valkenburg HA, Cats A. Evaluation of diagnostic criteria for ankylosing spondylitis. A proposal for modification of the New York criteria. Arthritis Rheum 1984;27(4):361–8.
5. Dougados M, van der Linden S, Juhlin R, et al. The European Spondylarthropathy Study Group preliminary criteria for the classification of spondylarthropathy. Arthritis Rheum 1991;34:1218–27.
6. Amor B, Dougados M, Mijiyawa M. Criteria for the classification of spondyloarthropathies. Rev Rhum Mal Osteoaric 1990;57:85–9.
7. Taylor W, Gladman D, Helliwell P, et al. Classification criteria for psoriatic arthritis: development of new criteria from a large international study. Arthritis Rheum 2006;54(8):2665–73.
8. Mease P, Khan M. Axial spondyloarthritis. St. Louis (MO): Elsevier; 2020. p. 294, 18 chapters.
9. Rudwaleit M, van der Heijde D, Landewe R, et al. The development of assessment of SpondyloArthritis International Society classification criteria for axial spondyloarthritis (part II): validation and final selection. Ann Rheum Dis 2009; 68(6):777–83.
10. Rudwaleit M, van der Heijde D, Landewe R, et al. The assessment of SpondyloArthritis International Society classification criteria for peripheral spondyloarthritis and for spondyloarthritis in general. Ann Rheum Dis 2011;70(1):25–31.
11. Raychaudhuri SP, Deodhar A. The classification and diagnostic criteria of ankylosing spondylitis. J Autoimmun 2014;48-49:128–33.
12. Sieper J, van der Heijde D, Landewe R, et al. New criteria for inflammatory back pain in patients with chronic back pain: a real patient exercise by experts from the assessment of SpondyloArthritis International Society (ASAS). Ann Rheum Dis 2009;68(6):784–8.
13. Rudwaleit M, van der Heijde D, Khan MA, et al. How to diagnose axial spondyloarthritis early. Ann Rheum Dis 2004;63(5):535–43.
14. van den Berg R, de Hooge M, Rudwaleit M, et al. ASAS modification of the Berlin algorithm for diagnosing axial spondyloarthritis: results from the SPondyloArthritis Caught Early (SPACE)-cohort and from the Assessment of SpondyloArthritis International Society (ASAS)-cohort. Ann Rheum Dis 2013;72(10):1646–53.
15. Rachakonda TD, Schupp CW, Armstrong AW. Psoriasis prevalence among adults in the United States. J Am Acad Dermatol 2014;70(3):512–6.
16. Mease PJ, Gladman DD, Papp KA, et al. Prevalence of rheumatologist-diagnosed psoriatic arthritis in patients with psoriasis in European/North American dermatology clinics. J Am Acad Dermatol 2013;69(5):729–35.
17. Ibrahim GH, Buch MH, Lawson C, et al. Evaluation of an existing screening tool for psoriatic arthritis in people with psoriasis and the development of a new instrument: the Psoriasis Epidemiology Screening Tool (PEST) questionnaire. Clin Exp Rheumatol 2009;27(3):469–74.

18. Ritchlin CT, Colbert RA, Gladman DD. Psoriatic arthritis. N Engl J Med 2017; 376(10):957–70.
19. Feld J, Chandran V, Haroon N, et al. Axial disease in psoriatic arthritis and anky-losing spondylitis: a critical comparison. Nat Rev Rheumatol 2018;14(6):363–71.
20. Feld J, Ye JY, Chandran V, et al. Is axial psoriatic arthritis distinct from ankylosing spondylitis with and without concomitant psoriasis? Rheumatology (Oxford) 2020; 59(6):1340–6.
21. Landau T, Cross R. Gastrointestinal tract and rheumatic disease. In: Hochberg MC, editor. Rheumatology. Philadelphia: Elsevier; 2018. p. 321–7.
22. Leirisalo-Repo M, Repo H. Reactive arthritis: clinical features and treatment. In: Hochberg MC, editor. Rheumatology. Philadelphia: Elsevier; 2018. p. 1113–20.
23. Ogdie A, Schwartzman S, Husni ME. Recognizing and managing comorbidities in psoriatic arthritis. Curr Opin Rheumatol 2015;27(2):118–26.
24. Mease PJ. Fibromyalgia, a missed comorbidity in spondyloarthritis: prevalence and impact on assessment and treatment. Curr Opin Rheumatol 2017;29(4):304–10.
25. Brown M, Xu H, Reveille J. Genetics of axial spondyloarthritis. In: Mease PJ, Khan M, editors. Axial spondyloarthritis. St Louis (MO): Elsevier; 2020. p. 67–86.
26. Sternes P, Brown M. The gut microbiome and ankylosing spondylitis. In: Mease PJ, Khan M, editors. Axial spondyloarthritis. St Louis (MO): Elsevier; 2020. p. 87–96.
27. Ciccia F, Srinath A, Zeng F, et al. Pathogenesis of ankylosing spondylitis. In: Mease PJ, Khan M, editors. Axial spondyloarthritis. St Louis (MO): Elsevier; 2020. p. 97–110.
28. Lories R. Bone pathophysiology in axial spondyloarthritis. In: Mease PJ, Khan M, editors. Axial spondyloarthritis. St Louis (MO): Elsevier; 2020. p. 111–20.
29. Lories RJ, McInnes IB. Primed for inflammation: enthesis-resident T cells. Nat Med 2012;18(7):1018–9.
30. Ozgocmen S. Nonpharmacologic management of axial spondyloarthritis. In: Mease PJ, Khan M, editors. Axial spondyloarthritis. St Louis (MO): Elsevier; 2020. p. 203–16.
31. Proft F, Poddubnyy D. Pharmacologic nonbiologic treatment of axial spondyloar-thritis. In: Mease PJ, Khan M, editors. Axial spondyloarthritis. St Louis (MO): Elsevier; 2020. p. 217–26.
32. Van den Bosch F, Carron P, Mease P. Biologic treatment of axial spondyloarthritis. In: Mease PJ, Khan M, editors. Axial spondyloarthritis. St Louis (MO): Elsevier; 2020. p. 227–42.
33. Kiwalkar S, Deodhar A, Sieper J. Treatment guidelines for axial spondyloarthritis. In: Axial spondyloarthritis. St Louis (MO): Elsevier; 2020. p. 243–58.
34. Mease PJ. Biologic therapy for psoriatic arthritis. Rheum Dis Clin North Am 2015; 41(4):723–38.
35. Mease PJ, Armstrong AW. Managing patients with psoriatic disease: the diag-nosis and pharmacologic treatment of psoriatic arthritis in patients with psoriasis. Drugs 2014;74(4):423–41.
36. Coates LC, Kavanaugh A, Mease PJ, et al. Group for research and assessment of psoriasis and psoriatic arthritis 2015 treatment recommendations for psoriatic arthritis. Arthritis Rheum 2016;68(5):1060–71.
37. Mease P. Emerging immunomodulatory therapies and new treatment paradigms for axial spondyloarthritis. Curr Rheumatol Rep 2019;21(7):35.
38. Ward MM, Deodhar A, Gensler LS, et al. 2019 update of the American College of Rheumatology/Spondylitis Association of America/Spondyloarthritis Research and Treatment Network Recommendations for the treatment of ankylosing spon-dylitis and nonradiographic axial spondyloarthritis. Arthritis Rheum 2019;71(10): 1599–613.

Pregnancy and Management in Women with Rheumatoid Arthritis, Systemic Lupus Erythematosus, and Obstetric Antiphospholipid Syndrome

Adela Castro-Gutierrez, MD, Kristen Young, MD,
Bonnie L. Bermas, MD*

KEYWORDS

- Pregnancy • Rheumatoid arthritis • Systemic lupus erythematosus • Obstetric APS

KEY POINTS

- Women with rheumatoid arthritis (RA) and systemic lupus erythematosus (SLE) are at risk for disease activity during pregnancy and adverse pregnancy outcomes.
- Pregnancies in women with RA and SLE do best if disease is under good control on pregnancy-compatible medications at the time of conception.
- Women with obstetric antiphospholipid syndrome (APS) are at risk for adverse pregnancy outcomes and need to be anticoagulated during pregnancy.
- Many but not all antirheumatic drugs can be continued during pregnancy.

Rheumatic diseases, such as rheumatoid arthritis (RA) and systemic lupus erythematosus (SLE), frequently affect women during their reproductive years. Moreover, women with antiphospholipid syndrome (APS) can have distinct obstetric complications that warrant monitoring and treatment. In this article, the authors discuss the impact of pregnancy on RA and SLE and the risk of adverse pregnancy outcome in these conditions. The evaluation and management of women with obstetric APS also are reviewed. In addition, the safety during pregnancy and lactation of the most commonly used medications in treating RA and SLE are discussed.

RHEUMATOID ARTHRITIS AND PREGNANCY

RA is a chronic inflammatory disease that commonly affects women of childbearing age. For many years, the teaching was that RA would go into remission in the vast

This article originally appeared in the Medical Clinics of North America, Volume 105, Issue 2, March 2021.
UT Southwestern Medical Center, 2001 Inwood Road, Dallas, TX 75390, USA
* Corresponding author.
E-mail address: Bonnie.Bermas@UTSouthwestern.edu

Rheum Dis Clin N Am 48 (2022) 523–535
https://doi.org/10.1016/j.rdc.2022.02.009
0889-857X/22/© 2022 Elsevier Inc. All rights reserved.

majority of patients and patients were taken off of their medications. More recently, data have shown that some patients with RA flare during pregnancy and good disease control is important prior to conception.

Fertility

Several studies have shown that women with RA have more difficulties conceiving, as indicated by a longer time to pregnancy (TTP), than those without RA.[1,2] Women with RA also have smaller-sized families than their peers.[3] Theories as to why there is increased infertility in these patients include physiologic changes and personal choices, due to either underlying disease or concerns regarding medications. There are unclear data regarding whether antimüllerian hormone (AMH), a marker of ovarian reserve, is abnormal in women with RA. Moreover, recent data suggest that levels of AMH in women with RA did not correlate with TTP or self-reported fertility.[4]

Pregnancy and Disease Flare

Slightly more than half of women with RA experience amelioration of disease during pregnancy. This improvement is associated with low disease activity at the time of conception and seronegativity (absence of a rheumatoid factor and/or anticitrulli-nated peptide antibodies). In one study, greater HLA disparity between mother and fetus was associated with successful pregnancy and induction of remission in patients with RA.[5] Additionally, some post-translational modifications like glycosyla-tion and galactosylation on immunoglobulins have been shown to affect their immuno-effector functions, which have been associated with favorable pregnancy outcomes.[6]

Assessing RA disease activity during pregnancy can be challenging particularly because the physiologic changes of pregnancy can have an impact on markers of RA disease activity, such as the erythrocyte sedimentation rate. In addition, joint pain and fluid retention are common in pregnancy and can be difficult to distinguish from an RA flare. Furthermore, not all scales used to assess disease activity are ac-curate during pregnancy; however, a study showed that using the Disease Activity Score in 28 joints calculated with C-reactive protein without global health scoring was useful in ascertaining clinical remission during pregnancy.[7] This study also found that patients with low disease activity were more likely to remain stable or go into remission during pregnancy whereas patients with high disease activity prior to pregnancy did not remit until the second and third trimesters. Other studies have shown that women with seronegative disease (absence of rheumatoid factor and anticitrullinated peptide antibodies) were more likely to improve and sustain low dis-ease activity during pregnancy.[8] In a study by van den Brandt and colleagues,[9] which included 75 pregnant patients with RA, it was found that most flares occurred within the first trimester and were associated with active disease prior to pregnancy along with discontinuation of therapies, such as tumor necrosis factor (TNF) inhibitors.

RA has been associated with adverse pregnancy outcomes, including intrauterine growth restriction (IUGR), premature rupture of membranes, and preterm delivery.[10] In a prospective study by de Man and colleagues,[11] which included patients from the Dutch health registry, higher RA disease activity as well as use of prednisone dur-ing pregnancy were associated with lower birth weights and increased cesarean sec-tions. Thus, if possible, RA pregnancies should be planned for periods of low disease activity.

SYSTEMIC LUPUS ERYTHEMATOSUS AND PREGNANCY

SLE is a multisystem disorder that occurs predominantly in reproductive-aged women. For many years, women with SLE were counseled to avoid pregnancy because of concerns regarding disease flare and adverse pregnancy outcome. More recently, data suggest that many women with women can have successful pregnancies if disease is under good control and planned.

Fertility

Women with SLE, like those with RA, have reduced family size.[12] Reduction in fertility is related to the use of cytotoxic medications, such as cyclophosphamide.[13] Disease itself, however, in the absence of such medications does not decrease fertility.[14] Data on AMH levels in SLE are conflicting, with some studies showing lower levels of AMH in SLE patients and other studies showing no difference once allowances were made for exposure to cytotoxic medications.[15,16] Secondary infertility, defined as spontaneous pregnancy loss, is increased in SLE patients but only in the setting of antiphospholipid antibodies (discussed later).

Pregnancy and Disease Flare

The advice, discussed previously, that women with SLE avoid pregnancy was based on concern for increase disease activity and adverse pregnancy outcome. Not all women with SLE, however, flare during pregnancy. Patients with a prior history of renal disease have a greater risk of disease flare during pregnancy. Primagravidas also have an increased risk of flare during pregnancy. Disease activity in the 6 months preceding pregnancy increases the risk of pregnancy-associated disease flare, with an estimated flare rate of 60% in women with active disease preconception. For this reason, SLE patients should be under good disease control with medications compatible with pregnancy for several months prior to conception. Disease manifestations during pregnancy are related to disease manifestations in the period of time preceding pregnancy.[17] For example, women who have skin manifestations in the prepregnancy period are more likely to have skin flares during pregnancy, whereas women with hematologic abnormalities prepregnancy are more likely to have hematologic abnormalities during a pregnancy flare.

Severe disease-related damage, such as significant renal insufficiency, pulmonary artery hypertension, and coronary artery disease, can cause severe maternal morbidity and, in some cases, mortality during pregnancy. Women with these conditions should be counseled about these risks prior to pursuing pregnancy.

Distinguishing lupus flare from preeclampsia can be challenging. Moreover, women with lupus have a higher incidence of preeclampsia than control populations. Active urine sediment, increasing double-stranded DNA titer, low complements, and leukopenia are suggestive of lupus flare whereas increasing liver-derived transaminases, uric acid levels, and proteinuria without an active sediment are more suggestive of preeclampsia. This distinction is important, however, because preeclampsia is an indication for emergent delivery, whereas SLE flare warrants aggressive immunosuppression.

SLE is associated with adverse pregnancy outcomes. A nationwide inpatient survey showed that women with SLE were more likely to have increased hypertension, IUGR, cesarean section rate, preeclampsia, and fetal death.[18] Although these data have improved somewhat over the past decade, the complication rate in SLE pregnancy still exceeds that in the general population.[19] The best prospective pregnancy study to date, the Predictors of Pregnancy Outcome: Biomarkers in Antiphospholipid

Syndrome and Systemic Lupus Erythematosus (PROMISSE) study, reported adverse pregnancy outcomes (fetal death, birth before 36 weeks' gestation, and small-for-gestational-age [SGA] infants) in 19% of women.[20] Primagravidas, lupus anticoagulant (LA), antihypertensive medication, and active disease all predict poor outcome. Overall, however, the complication rate was low and somewhat reflective of the low-disease-activity SLE patient population.

Patients with SLE should be on pregnancy-compatible medication to maintain low disease activity prior to pregnancy. Several studies have shown that hydroxychloroquine during pregnancy improves outcome.[21] Nonetheless, disappointingly, claims data suggest that only a small percentage of patients are adherent with their hydroxychloroquine during pregnancy.[22]

OBSTETRIC ANTIPHOSPHOLIPID SYNDROME

APS is a systemic autoimmune disorder associated with venous and arterial thrombosis and obstetric complications. It exists as primary APS, secondary or related to underlying autoimmune disease, or obstetric APS. This discussion focuses on obstetric APS. Clinically, obstetric APS is defined as pregnancy loss or delivery at less than 34 weeks of gestation because of preeclampsia or evidence of placental insufficiency, 1 or more unexplained fetal deaths at greater than 10 weeks' gestation, or 3 or greater unexplained spontaneous pregnancy losses before 10 weeks of gestation. Clinical manifestations must be associated with laboratory criteria, including the presence of persistent LA, anticardiolipin antibody (aCL), or anti–beta-2 glycoprotein I.[23] The LA and triple-positivity LA, aCL, and anti–beta-2 glycoprotein I are associated most commonly with adverse pregnancy outcome.[24,25] The significance of other antiphospholipid antibodies, such as antiphosphatidylserine /prothrombin antibodies, is unproved, although 1 study showed the presence of these antibodies in 86% of patients with APS.[26] In addition to fetal loss, women with obstetric APS have higher incidence of preeclampsia, eclampsia, and HELLP syndrome. Adverse fetal outcomes include prematurity and IUGR. Women who have a history of unexplained preeclampsia, premature infants, and recurrent pregnancy loss should be evaluated for antiphospholipid antibodies, including an LA, aCL and anti–beta-2 glycoprotein I.

Management

Women with obstetric APS required anticoagulation.[27] Although unfractionated heparin can be used, low-molecular-weight heparin (LMWH) is preferred because steady-state levels are easier to maintain. In women with only obstetric manifestations, prophylactic-dose LMWH can be used whereas those women with thrombotic manifestations as well need therapeutic anticoagulation during pregnancy. Warfarin is contraindicated during pregnancy. There are insufficient data to conclude the efficacy of the direct oral anticoagulants during pregnancy in APS or the safety of these medications during pregnancy. In addition to LMWH, patients should be treated with a baby aspirin.[28]

MANAGEMENT OF RHEUMATOID ARTHRITIS AND SYSTEMIC LUPUS ERYTHEMATOSUS DURING PREGNANCY

The key component of management of RA and SLE during pregnancy is having patients under good control on medications compatible with pregnancy (**Table 1**) prior to conception. Importantly, patients ideally should be managed by a team of

Table 1
Medication compatibility with pregnancy and lactation

Pregnancy Risk	Pregnancy	Lactation
Compatible	Monitor mother for hypertension	Compatible
Hydroxychloroquine		Compatible
Sulfasalazine		Compatible
Azathioprine		Compatible
Cyclosporine		Compatible
Tacrolimus		Compatible
Low-dose aspirin		
Some risk	Stop by 30 weeks—risk of patent	Preference for short-acting
NSAIDs	ductus arteriosus	>20 mg/d discard
Glucocorticoids	Keep dose as low as possible	breastmilk for 40
TNF-α blockers	Discontinue third trimester[a]	following dose
Rituximab	Discontinue at conception	Compatible
Belimumab	Discontinue at conception	Compatible
Abatacept	Discontinue at conception	Compatible
Tocilizumab	Discontinue at conception	Compatible
		Compatible
Avoid during pregnancy	Stop 1–3 mo before conception	Incompatible
Methotrexate	Levels should be undetectable	Incompatible
Thalidomide		Incompatible
Leflunomide		Incompatible
Mycophenolate mofetil		Incompatible
Cyclophosphamide		
Insufficient data		Avoid during lactation—
Tofacitinib		small molecules readily
Baricitinib		pass into breast milk

[a] Certolizumab may be continued throughout pregnancy. Other TNF-α blockers can possibly continue through pregnancy if disease activity is high.

providers, including those familiar with rheumatic diseases and skilled in maternal fetal medicine.

MEDICATIONS DURING PREGNANCY AND LACTATION

Data on medication safety during pregnancy and lactation often are limited. For many years, providers relied on the US Food and Drug Administration (FDA) use in pregnancy ratings A, B, C, D and X. These ratings were inappropriately interpreted as a grading system, when in actuality they reflected the amount of available data regarding a specific drug's safety during pregnancy. In order to mitigate these shortcomings, the FDA instituted the Pregnancy and Lactation Labeling rule in 2015 an attempt to provide clinicians with comprehensive and up-to-date information regarding medication safety during pregnancy and lactation in order to inform decision making.[29] Nonetheless, the information provided within the new system leaves much of the interpretation of the data up to the individual clinician. Fortunately, over the past few years, several professional organizations, including the British Society for Rheumatology, the European League Against Rheumatism, and more recently the American College of Rheumatology, have published guidelines regarding use of medications during pregnancy and lactation.[30–32]

Medications that are Compatible during Pregnancy and Lactation

Hydroxychloroquine is the mainstay of therapy for women with SLE and connective tissue disease (diseases that have features of rheumatic disorders but who cannot be definitively categorized). This medication has no teratogenic risk when taken during pregnancy. Moreover, ample evidence suggested continuation of hydroxychloroquine during pregnancy improves outcome. In a retrospective study of 257 pregnancies from the Johns Hopkins Lupus Cohort, discontinuation of hydroxychloroquine was associated with increased risk of lupus flare.[21] This medication is compatible with breastfeeding.[33]

Sulfasalazine is used to manage joint inflammation in persons with RA and, less commonly, SLE. A large meta-analysis did not show any increase in fetal anomalies after in utero exposure.[34] Although there has been 1 report of a breastfeeding infant who had bloody diarrhea after his mother was given sulfasalazine, this medication is considered compatible with lactation.[35]

The immunosuppressive agents azathioprine, cyclosporine, and more recently tacrolimus are used as immunosuppressive agents in women with SLE, in particular for induction and maintenance therapy for lupus renal disease. There is ample literature from the transplant population that these medications do not increase the risk for congenital anomalies.[11,12,36–40] These medications are compatible with pregnancy and with nursing.[32]

Aspirin does not appear to be teratogenic in humans. One large study of 5128 pregnancies in which there was in utero aspirin exposure did not show increased congenital anomalies.[41] Moreover, this medication has been part of the regimen for the management of obstetric APS.[42] Moreover, data suggest that baby aspirin may decrease the risk of preeclampsia.[43] The American College of Obstetricians and Gynecologists recommends the use of this medication in persons with disorders, such as SLE and APS, because these patients may have an increased risk for preeclampsia. Aspirin is compatible with breastfeeding.

Medications with Some Risk for use during Pregnancy and Lactation

Glucocorticoids frequently are used to manage disease flares in a variety of rheumatic diseases. The nonfluorinated medications used most commonly to manage rheumatic diseases are prednisone and prednisolone. These medications do not readily cross the placenta.[44] Although 1 meta-analysis suggested that glucocorticoids increased the risk of cleft palate formation 2-fold after in utero exposure,[45] a large Danish cohort study that examined 51,973 first-trimester glucocorticoid exposure failed to show any increase risk of cleft lip and/or palate formation.[46] Although there does not appear to be an increased risk of congenital anomaly in infants exposed to this medication in utero, these medications increase the risk of preeclampsia, preterm premature rupture of the membranes, gestational diabetes, hypertension, and SGA infants. Prednisone and prednisolone are compatible with breastfeeding; however, it is recommended in women who are using doses of greater than 20 mg a day discard breast milk for the first 4 hours after dosing.[30]

Non-steroidal anti-inflammatory drugs (NSAIDs) and cyclooxygenase (COX-2) inhibitors are used to manage pain and inflammation in individuals with RA and SLE. Although NSAIDs do not increase the risk of congenital anomalies,[47] 1 meta-analysis found the risk of ductal closure to be 15-fold higher in women exposed to indomethacin during the third trimester of pregnancy.[48] There are conflicting data on whether nonsteroidal use during the first trimester increases the risk for spontaneous miscarriage. One large case-control study suggested that there was an increased odds ratio for miscarriage in pregnancies exposed to NSAIDs[49]; however, another study of more than 65,000 pregnancies did not show any increased risk for spontaneous abortion after NSAID exposure.[50] Data suggest that NSAIDs are compatible with nursing, although there is a slight preference for ibuprofen given its short half-life. There are insufficient data to evaluate pregnancy safety of COX-2 inhibitors.

Although initially there were concerns that the TNF-α blockers may contribute to the vertebral defects, anal atresia, cardiac defects, tracheoesophageal fistula, renal anomalies, and limb abnormalities (VACTERL) syndrome, subsequent data have not supported this finding.[51,52] There is ample evidence that TNF-α blockers not only are compatible with pregnancy but also are important for good disease control of inflammatory arthritis that contributes to improved pregnancy outcome. There are no clear-cut recommendations for when TNF-α blockers should be discontinued, but several professional organizations recommend discontinuing these medications during the third trimester.[30–32] This recommendation is based on reducing the risk of immunosuppression of neonates.[53] In patients with active disease, however, continuing these drugs through delivery can be considered. Certolizumab is a TNF-α blocker that is pegylated and does not cross the placenta in any significant amount.[54] This medication may be continued throughout pregnancy. The TNF-α blockers all are large molecules and little drug gets transferred into breast milk. Lactating women can take these medications.

The biologics, such as rituximab, belimumab, tocilizumab, and abatacept, do not effectively transfer to the placenta until 12 weeks to 15 weeks of gestation. Although data are limited, studies in which belimumab and rituximab were continued through early pregnancy did not show any significant safety signals.[55,56] Current recommendations by several professional organizations are that these medications can be included until conception.

MEDICATIONS THAT ARE CONTRAINDICATED IN PREGNANCY

The medications leflunomide, methotrexate, mycophenolate mofetil, and cyclophosphamide are contraindicated during pregnancy. Leflunomide is an antimetabolite that inhibits dihydroorotate dehydrogenase. Its major metabolite, teriflunomide, is detectable in the serum for up to 2 years. This drug is major teratogen in animals and for this reason is contraindicated during pregnancy.[57] Human data are more reassuring because there has no pattern of congenital anomalies reported after preconception and early pregnancy exposure to leflunomide[58]; nonetheless, this medication should be discontinued prior to conception and blood levels should be undetectable. The latter can be achieved by cholestyramine washout or by discontinuing the medication for 2 years prior to conception. Methotrexate is both teratogenic and abortogenic and women should discontinue this medication 1 months to 3 months prior to conception.[59,60] Mycophenolate mofetil causes a higher than expected rate of congenital anomalies and should be discontinued 6 weeks prior to conception.[61] Likewise, cyclophosphamide is teratogenic and should be avoided during pregnancy.[62] Cyclophosphamide, however, has been used in the late pregnancy for cancers and lupus nephritis with no minimal risk to the fetus.[63,64] None of these medications is compatible with lactation.

Insufficient Data

Although 1 small case series did not suggest there were safety concerns after in utero exposure to tofacitinib,[65] there are insufficient data to conclude safety of the small molecules tofacitinib and baricitinib during pregnancy. These molecules are small and readily pass into breast milk and, therefore, should be avoided in lactating women.

SUMMARY

RA, SLE, and APS are associated with risk of disease activity during pregnancy and pregnancy complications. Many but not all RA patients go into remission during pregnancy. Active disease prior to conception and discontinuation of medications, in particular TNF-α blockers, portend greater disease activity during pregnancy. RA pregnancies in which disease is poorly controlled have higher risks of adverse pregnancy outcome, including preeclampsia, prematurity, and SGA infants. SLE patients who have a prior history of lupus nephritis are particularly vulnerable to increased disease activity during pregnancy. This, is turn, is associated with adverse pregnancy outcome, including preterm premature rupture of the membranes, SGA infants, and preeclampsia. Patients with SLE should be maintained on their hydroxychloroquine during pregnancy, and conception should be deferred until disease is under good control with pregnancy-compatible medication for several months. Comanagement with a maternal fetal specialist is crucial. Obstetric APS carries risks of adverse pregnancy outcome. Anticoagulation with fractionated or unfractionated heparin along with baby aspirin mitigates this risk. Although not all medications can be used during pregnancy, many medications used to treat RA and SLE can be continued. Hydroxychloroquine, sulfasalazine, and the immunosuppressive agents azathioprine, cyclosporine, and tacrolimus can be continued throughout pregnancy and during lactation. NSAIDs can be used but must be stopped by the third trimester due to the risk of patent ductus arteriosus. Glucocorticoids can be used but do carry risks of comorbidity. The TNF-α blockers can be continued to the third trimester of pregnancy and on a case-by-case basis consideration can be given to consider continuing them through delivery. Biologics, such as rituximab, belimumab, abatacept, and tocilizumab, may be continued through conception. Leflunomide, methotrexate, thalidomide, mycophenolate mofetil, and cyclophosphamide are contraindicated during pregnancy. There are insufficient data to conclude the safety of the small molecules during pregnancy and lactation; therefore, they should be discontinued prior to conception. With good disease control and a team approach with both a rheumatology provider and, if possible, a maternal-fetal-medicine provider, many RA, SLE, and APS patients can anticipate a good pregnancy outcome.

CLINICS CARE POINTS

- Women with RA and SLE should have their disease under good control on pregnancy-compatible medications and observed for several months prior to attempting conception.
- Methotrexate, thalidomide, leflunomide, mycophenolate mofetil, and cyclophosphamide are teratogenic, and these medications should be avoided in pregnant and lactating women.
- Women with SLE should be encouraged to take hydroxychloroquine during pregnancy because this medication improves outcomes for mother and fetus.
- Women with APS (obstetric and clotting manifestations) should be anticoagulated during pregnancy.

REFERENCES

1. Jawaheer D, Zhu JL, Nohr EA, et al. Time to pregnancy among women with rheumatoid arthritis. Arthritis Rheum 2011;63(6):1517–21. Available at: http://doi.wiley.com/10.1002/art.30327.
2. Brouwer J, Fleurbaaij R, Hazes JMW, et al. Subfertility in Women With Rheumatoid Arthritis and the Outcome of Fertility Assessments. Arthritis Care Res (Hoboken) 2017;69(8):1142–9. Available at: http://www.ncbi.nlm.nih.gov/pubmed/27723275.
3. Provost M, Eaton JL, Clowse MEB. Fertility and infertility in rheumatoid arthritis. Curr Opin Rheumatol 2014;26(3):308–14. Available at: http://journals.lww.com/00002281-201405000-00011.
4. Eudy AM, McDaniel G, Hurd WW, et al. Fertility and Ovarian Reserve among Women with Rheumatoid Arthritis. J Rheumatol 2019;46(5):455–9. Available at: http://www.jrheum.org/lookup/doi/10.3899/jrheum.180176.
5. Zrour SH, Boumiza R, Sakly N, et al. The impact of pregnancy on rheumatoid arthritis outcome: the role of maternofetal HLA class II disparity. Joint Bone Spine 2010;77(1):36–40. Available at: http://www.ncbi.nlm.nih.gov/pubmed/20031464.
6. Förger F, Villiger PM. Immunological adaptations in pregnancy that modulate rheumatoid arthritis disease activity. Nat Rev Rheumatol 2020;16(2):113–22. Available at: http://www.nature.com/articles/s41584-019-0351-2.
7. de Man YA, Dolhain RJEM, van de Geijn FE, et al. Disease activity of rheumatoid arthritis during pregnancy: results from a nationwide prospective study. Arthritis Rheum 2008;59(9):1241–8. Available at: http://www.ncbi.nlm.nih.gov/pubmed/18759316.
8. Förger F, Vallbracht I, Helmke K, et al. Pregnancy mediated improvement of rheumatoid arthritis. Swiss Med Wkly 2012;. http://doi.emh.ch/smw.2012.13644.
9. van den Brandt S, Zbinden A, Baeten D, et al. Risk factors for flare and treatment of disease flares during pregnancy in rheumatoid arthritis and axial spondyloarthritis patients. Arthritis Res Ther 2017;19(1):64. Available at: http://www.ncbi.nlm.nih.gov/pubmed/28320445.
10. Kishore S, Mittal V, Majithia V. Obstetric outcomes in women with rheumatoid arthritis: Results from Nationwide Inpatient Sample Database 2003–2011☆. Semin Arthritis Rheum 2019;49(2):236–40. Available at: https://linkinghub.elsevier.com/retrieve/pii/S0049017218306334.
11. de Man YA, Hazes JMW, van der Heide H, et al. Association of higher rheumatoid arthritis disease activity during pregnancy with lower birth weight: Results of a national prospective study. Arthritis Rheum 2009;60(11):3196–206. Available at: http://doi.wiley.com/10.1002/art.24914.
12. Ekblom-Kullberg S, Kautiainen H, Alha P, et al. Reproductive health in women with systemic lupus erythematosus compared to population controls. Scand J Rheumatol 2009;38(5):375–80. Available at: http://www.tandfonline.com/doi/full/10.1080/03009740902763099.
13. McDermott EM, Powell RJ. Incidence of ovarian failure in systemic lupus erythematosus after treatment with pulse cyclophosphamide. Ann Rheum Dis 1996;55(4):224–9. Available at: http://www.ncbi.nlm.nih.gov/pubmed/8733438.
14. Hickman RA, Gordon C. Causes and management of infertility in systemic lupus erythematosus. Rheumatology 2011;50(9):1551–8. Available at: https://academic.oup.com/rheumatology/article-lookup/doi/10.1093/rheumatology/ker105.
15. Gao H, Ma J, Wang X, et al. Preliminary study on the changes of ovarian reserve, menstruation, and lymphocyte subpopulation in systemic lupus erythematosus

(SLE) patients of childbearing age. Lupus 2018;27(3):445–53. Available at: http://journals.sagepub.com/doi/10.1177/0961203317726378.

16. Di Mario C, Petricca L, Gigante MR, et al. Anti-Müllerian hormone serum levels in systemic lupus erythematosus patients: Influence of the disease severity and therapy on the ovarian reserve. Endocrine 2019;63(2):369–75. Available at: http://link.springer.com/10.1007/s12020-018-1783-1.

17. Tedeschi SK, Massarotti E, Guan H, et al. Specific systemic lupus erythematosus disease manifestations in the six months prior to conception are associated with similar disease manifestations during pregnancy. Lupus 2015;24(12):1283–92. Available at: http://journals.sagepub.com/doi/10.1177/0961203315586455.

18. Chakravarty EF, Nelson L, Krishnan E. Obstetric hospitalizations in the United States for women with systemic lupus erythematosus and rheumatoid arthritis. Arthritis Rheum 2006;54(3):899–907. Available at: http://www.ncbi.nlm.nih.gov/pubmed/16508972.

19. Mehta B, Luo Y, Xu J, et al. Trends in Maternal and Fetal Outcomes Among Pregnant Women With Systemic Lupus Erythematosus in the United States. Ann Intern Med 2019;171(3):164. Available at: https://annals.org/aim/fullarticle/2737824/trends-maternal-fetal-outcomes-among-pregnant-women-systemic-lupus-erythematosus.

20. Buyon JP, Kim MY, Guerra MM, et al. Predictors of Pregnancy Outcomes in Patients With Lupus. Ann Intern Med 2015;163(3):153. Available at: http://annals.org/article.aspx?doi=10.7326/M14-2235.

21. Clowse MEB, Magder L, Witter F, et al. Hydroxychloroquine in lupus pregnancy. Arthritis Rheum 2006;54(11):3640–7. Available at: http://doi.wiley.com/10.1002/art.22159.

22. Bermas BL, Kim SC, Huybrechts K, et al. Trends in use of hydroxychloroquine during pregnancy in systemic lupus erythematosus patients from 2001 to 2015. Lupus 2018;27(6):1012–7. Available at: http://www.degruyter.com/view/j/cclm.2018.56.issue-4/cclm-2017-0502/cclm-2017-0502.xml.

23. MIYAKIS S, LOCKSHIN MD, ATSUMI T, et al. International consensus statement on an update of the classification criteria for definite antiphospholipid syndrome (APS). J Thromb Haemost 2006;4(2):295–306. Available at: http://doi.wiley.com/10.1111/j.1538-7836.2006.01753.x.

24. Yelnik CM, Laskin CA, Porter TF, et al. Lupus anticoagulant is the main predictor of adverse pregnancy outcomes in aPL-positive patients: validation of PROMISSE study results. Lupus Sci Med 2016;3(1):e000131. Available at: http://lupus.bmj.com/lookup/doi/10.1136/lupus-2015-000131.

25. Lazzaroni M-G, Fredi M, Andreoli L, et al. Triple Antiphospholipid (aPL) Antibodies Positivity Is Associated With Pregnancy Complications in aPL Carriers: A Multicenter Study on 62 Pregnancies. Front Immunol 2019;10:1948. Available at: https://www.frontiersin.org/article/10.3389/fimmu.2019.01948/full.

26. Shi H, Zheng H, Yin Y-F, et al. Antiphosphatidylserine/prothrombin antibodies (aPS/PT) as potential diagnostic markers and risk predictors of venous thrombosis and obstetric complications in antiphospholipid syndrome. Clin Chem Lab Med 2018;56(4):614–24. Available at: http://www.degruyter.com/view/j/cclm.2018.56.issue-4/cclm-2017-0502/cclm-2017-0502.xml.

27. Kutteh WH, Hinote CD. Antiphospholipid Antibody Syndrome. Obstet Gynecol Clin North Am 2014;41(1):113–32. Available at: https://linkinghub.elsevier.com/retrieve/pii/S0889854513000910.

28. Gerardi MC, Fernandes MA, Tincani A, et al. Obstetric Anti-phospholipid Syndrome: State of the Art. Curr Rheumatol Rep 2018;20(10):59. Available at: http://link.springer.com/10.1007/s11926-018-0772-y.

29. Bermas BL, Tassinari M, Clowse M, et al. The new FDA labeling rule: impact on prescribing rheumatological medications during pregnancy. Rheumatology (Oxford) 2018;57(suppl_5):v2–8. Available at: http://www.ncbi.nlm.nih.gov/pubmed/30137587.

30. Flint J, Panchal S, Hurrell A, et al. BSR and BHPR guideline on prescribing drugs in pregnancy and breastfeeding—Part II: analgesics and other drugs used in rheumatology practice: Table 1. Rheumatology 2016;55(9):1698–702. Available from: https://academic.oup.com/rheumatology/article-lookup/doi/10.1093/rheumatology/kev405.

31. Götestam Skorpen C, Hoeltzenbein M, Tincani A, et al. The EULAR points to consider for use of antirheumatic drugs before pregnancy, and during pregnancy and lactation. Ann Rheum Dis 2016;75(5):795–810. Available at: http://ard.bmj.com/lookup/doi/10.1136/annrheumdis-2015-208840.

32. Sammaritano LR, Bermas BL, Chakravarty EE, et al. 2020 American College of Rheumatology Guideline for the Management of Reproductive Health in Rheumatic and Musculoskeletal Diseases. Arthritis Rheumatol 2020;72(4):529–56. Available at: http://www.ncbi.nlm.nih.gov/pubmed/32090480.

33. Section on Breastfeeding. Breastfeeding and the use of human milk. Pediatrics 2012;129(3):e827–41.   Available   at: http://www.ncbi.nlm.nih.gov/pubmed/22371471.

34. Rahimi R, Nikfar S, Rezaie A, et al. Pregnancy outcome in women with inflammatory bowel disease following exposure to 5-aminosalicylic acid drugs: a meta-analysis. Reprod Toxicol 2008;25(2):271–5. Available at: http://www.ncbi.nlm.nih.gov/pubmed/18242053.

35. Branski D, Kerem E, Gross-Kieselstein E, et al. Bloody diarrhea–a possible complication of sulfasalazine transferred through human breast milk. J Pediatr Gastroenterol Nutr 1986;5(2):316–7. Available at: http://www.ncbi.nlm.nih.gov/pubmed/2870147.

36. Goldstein LH, Dolinsky G, Greenberg R, et al. Pregnancy outcome of women exposed to azathioprine during pregnancy. Birth Defects Res A Clin Mol Teratol 2007;79(10):696–701.   Available   at: http://www.ncbi.nlm.nih.gov/pubmed/17847119.

37. Haugen G, Fauchald P, Sødal G, et al. Pregnancy outcome in renal allograft recipients in Norway. The importance of immunosuppressive drug regimen and health status before pregnancy. Acta Obstet Gynecol Scand 1994;73(7):541–6. Available at: http://www.ncbi.nlm.nih.gov/pubmed/8079604.

38. Radomski JS, Ahlswede BA, Jarrell BE, et al. Outcomes of 500 pregnancies in 335 female kidney, liver, and heart transplant recipients. Transplant Proc 1995;27(1):1089–90. Available at: http://www.ncbi.nlm.nih.gov/pubmed/7878816.

39. Bar Oz B, Hackman R, Einarson T, et al. Pregnancy outcome after cyclosporine therapy during pregnancy: a meta-analysis. Transplantation 2001;71(8):1051–5. Available at: http://www.ncbi.nlm.nih.gov/pubmed/11374400.

40. Kainz A, Harabacz I, Cowlrick IS, et al. Review of the course and outcome of 100 pregnancies in 84 women treated with tacrolimus. Transplantation 2000;70(12):1718–21. Available at: http://www.ncbi.nlm.nih.gov/pubmed/11152103.

41. Slone D, Siskind V, Heinonen OP, et al. Aspirin and congenital malformations. Lancet   1976;1(7974):1373–5.   Available   at: http://www.ncbi.nlm.nih.gov/pubmed/59014.

42. Cowchock S. Treatment of antiphospholipid syndrome in pregnancy. Lupus 1998;7(Suppl 2):S95–7. Available at: http://www.ncbi.nlm.nih.gov/pubmed/9814682.

43. Askie LM, Duley L, Henderson-Smart DJ, et al, PARIS Collaborative Group. Anti-platelet agents for prevention of pre-eclampsia: a meta-analysis of individual patient data. Lancet 2007;369(9575):1791–8. Available at: http://www.ncbi.nlm.nih.gov/pubmed/17512048.

44. Blanford AT, Murphy BE. In vitro metabolism of prednisolone, dexamethasone, betamethasone, and cortisol by the human placenta. Am J Obstet Gynecol 1977;127(3):264–7. Available at: http://www.ncbi.nlm.nih.gov/pubmed/835623.

45. Park-Wyllie L, Mazzotta P, Pastuszak A, et al. Birth defects after maternal exposure to corticosteroids: prospective cohort study and meta-analysis of epidemiological studies. Teratology 2000;62(6):385–92. Available at: http://www.ncbi.nlm.nih.gov/pubmed/11091630.

46. Hviid A, Mølgaard-Nielsen D. Corticosteroid use during pregnancy and risk of orofacial clefts. CMAJ 2011;183(7):796–804. Available at: http://www.ncbi.nlm.nih.gov/pubmed/21482652.

47. Schoenfeld A, Bar Y, Merlob P, et al. NSAIDs: maternal and fetal considerations. Am J Reprod Immunol 1992;28(3–4):141–7. Available at: http://www.ncbi.nlm.nih.gov/pubmed/1285865.

48. Koren G, Florescu A, Costei AM, et al. Nonsteroidal antiinflammatory drugs during third trimester and the risk of premature closure of the ductus arteriosus: a meta-analysis. Ann Pharmacother 2006;40(5):824–9. Available at: http://www.ncbi.nlm.nih.gov/pubmed/16638921.

49. Nakhai-Pour HR, Broy P, Sheehy O, et al. Use of nonaspirin nonsteroidal anti-inflammatory drugs during pregnancy and the risk of spontaneous abortion. CMAJ 2011;183(15):1713–20. Available at: http://www.ncbi.nlm.nih.gov/pubmed/21896698.

50. Daniel S, Koren G, Lunenfeld E, et al. Fetal exposure to nonsteroidal anti-inflammatory drugs and spontaneous abortions. CMAJ 2014;186(5):E177–82. Available at: http://www.ncbi.nlm.nih.gov/pubmed/24491470.

51. Carter JD, Ladhani A, Ricca LR, et al. A safety assessment of tumor necrosis factor antagonists during pregnancy: a review of the Food and Drug Administration database. J Rheumatol 2009;36(3):635–41. Available at: http://www.ncbi.nlm.nih.gov/pubmed/19132789.

52. Weber-Schoendorfer C, Oppermann M, Wacker E, et al. Pregnancy outcome after TNF-α inhibitor therapy during the first trimester: a prospective multicentre cohort study. Br J Clin Pharmacol 2015;80(4):727–39. Available at: http://www.ncbi.nlm.nih.gov/pubmed/25808588.

53. Pham-Huy A, Sadarangani M, Huang V, et al. From mother to baby: antenatal exposure to monoclonal antibody biologics. Expert Rev Clin Immunol 2019;15(3):221–9. Available at: https://www.tandfonline.com/doi/full/10.1080/1744666X.2019.1561282.

54. Clowse MEB, Wolf DC, Förger F, et al. Pregnancy Outcomes in Subjects Exposed to Certolizumab Pegol. J Rheumatol 2015;42(12):2270–8. Available at: http://www.ncbi.nlm.nih.gov/pubmed/26523031.

55. Peart E, Clowse MEB. Systemic lupus erythematosus and pregnancy outcomes. Curr Opin Rheumatol 2014;26(2):118–23. Available at: http://journals.lww.com/00002281-201403000-00004.

56. Chakravarty EF, Murray ER, Kelman A, et al. Pregnancy outcomes after maternal exposure to rituximab. Blood 2011;117(5):1499–506. Available at: http://www.ncbi.nlm.nih.gov/pubmed/21098742.

57. De Santis M. Paternal and maternal exposure to leflunomide: pregnancy and neonatal outcome. Ann Rheum Dis 2005;64(7):1096–7. Available at: http://ard. bmj.com/cgi/doi/10.1136/ard.2004.030254.

58. Cassina M, Johnson DL, Robinson LK, et al. Pregnancy outcome in women exposed to leflunomide before or during pregnancy. Arthritis Rheum 2012; 64(7):2085–94. Available at: http://www.ncbi.nlm.nih.gov/pubmed/22307734.

59. Hoppe DE, Bekkar BE, Nager CW. Single-dose systemic methotrexate for the treatment of persistent ectopic pregnancy after conservative surgery. Obstet Gynecol 1994;83(1):51–4. Available at: http://www.ncbi.nlm.nih.gov/pubmed/ 8272308.

60. Bawle EV, Conard JV, Weiss L. Adult and two children with fetal methotrexate syndrome. Teratology 1998;57(2):51–5. Available at: http://www.ncbi.nlm.nih.gov/ pubmed/9562676.

61. Hoeltzenbein M, Elefant E, Vial T, et al. Teratogenicity of mycophenolate confirmed in a prospective study of the European Network of Teratology Information Services. Am J Med Genet A 2012;158A(3):588–96. Available at: http://www. ncbi.nlm.nih.gov/pubmed/22319001.

62. Toledo TM, Harper RC, Moser RH. Fetal effects during cyclophosphamide and irradiation therapy. Ann Intern Med 1971;74(1):87–91. Available at: http://www. ncbi.nlm.nih.gov/pubmed/5539280.

63. Ring AE, Smith IE, Jones A, et al. Chemotherapy for Breast Cancer During Pregnancy: An 18-Year Experience From Five London Teaching Hospitals. J Clin Oncol 2005;23(18):4192–7. Available at: http://ascopubs.org/doi/10.1200/JCO. 2005.03.038.

64. Közdemir HK, Yücel AE, Künefeci G, et al. Cyclophosphamide therapy in a serious case of lupus nephritis during pregnancy. Lupus 2001;10(11):818–20. Available at: http://journals.sagepub.com/doi/10.1177/096120330101001110.

65. Clowse MEB, Feldman SR, Isaacs JD, et al. Pregnancy Outcomes in the Tofacitinib Safety Databases for Rheumatoid Arthritis and Psoriasis. Drug Saf 2016; 39(8):755–62. Available at: http://www.ncbi.nlm.nih.gov/pubmed/27282428.

Rheumatoid Arthritis
Early Diagnosis and Treatment

John J. Cush, MD

KEYWORDS

- Early rheumatoid arthritis • Referral • Rheumatoid factor

KEY POINTS

- Rheumatoid arthritis is not a laboratory diagnosis.
- Additive, symmetric polyarthritis of small and large joints.
- Do not wait for classicate features (nodules, erosions, deformity).
- Only use corticosteroids as bridge therapy while waiting for DMARDs to be effective.
- Start DMARD therapy and refer as soon as the diagnosis is made.

Rheumatoid arthritis (RA) is a chronic, progressive inflammatory disorder that manifests as a symmetric polyarthritis of small and large joints that may lead to joint and periarticular structural damage and the consequences of systemic inflammation.[1] Recent advances have resulted in better diagnostic criteria, improved serologic testing, novel new drugs, and better guidelines to manage patients with RA. Yet, there are challenges and unmet needs that frustrate patients and physicians alike, including:

- Delays in referral and early diagnosis
- Misuse of serologic testing
- Misconceptions about seronegative RA
- Faulty beliefs that RA drugs are more dangerous than RA itself

RA can be deadly. Many studies have shown that patients with RA live 6 to 11 fewer years than people without RA. This is especially true in women, those with seropositive RA, and those with active or recalcitrant RA. Patients with RA are at greater risk[2,3] to develop the following:

- Functional impairment and disability.
- Serious infections: Pneumonia is the number one cause of infectious death in RA. This risk is largely driven by: (1) the severity of RA, (2) steroid use (glucocorticoids are acutely wonderful, but they are chronically hazardous), (3) breakdown of skin

This article originally appeared in the Medical Clinics of North America, Volume 105, Issue 2, March 2021.
Rheumatic Disease Division, The University of Texas Southwestern Medical School, 9900 North Central Expressway, Suite 550, Dallas, TX 75231, USA
E-mail address: jjcush@gmail.com
Twitter: @rheumnow (J.J.C.)

Rheum Dis Clin N Am 48 (2022) 537–547
https://doi.org/10.1016/j.rdc.2022.02.010
0889-857X/22/

(from open ulcers, wounds, and major surgery), and (4) antirheumatic drugs. Although methotrexate (MTX), immunosuppressives, and biologics are often blamed for infectious events, they are only contributory after all of the afore mentioned have upped the risk of infection.

- Lymphoma and cancer: Cancer is one of the top three causes of death in RA. Patients with RA have a higher risk of non-Hodgkin lymphoma, lung cancer, and skin cancers; but have a lower risk of colon and breast cancer. This risk is largely independent of therapies, as and the cancer risk is predominantly driven by chronic inflammation.
- Cardiovascular (CV) death: CV disease is a consequence of chronic uncontrolled inflammation that affects the vasculature and myocardium. The CV risk in RA is further compounded by nonsteroidal anti-inflammatory drug use, weight gain, sedentary lifestyle, and other comorbidities. Control of inflammation and RA activity by prolonged treatment with MTX or other aggressive therapies (eg, biologics) lowers the CV event and death rate in RA.
- Chronic lung disease: Chronic lung disease in RA denotes those who are severe and have a higher mortality risk, especially for lung-related deaths.[4] Up to 20% of patients have chronic interstitial lung disease (ILD) and chronic lung disease is a major risk factor for infections, pneumonia, and death in RA.
- Extra-articular manifestations: These seem to also be a consequence of chronic inflammation and include such manifestations as rheumatoid nodules, Sjögren syndrome (dry eyes, dry mouth), rheumatoid vasculitis, rheumatoid lung, inflammatory eye disease (scleritis), Felty syndrome, amyloidosis, and neuropathy. These occur with more severe disease; seropositivity; and destructive, erosive arthritis.
- Surgery and complications of surgery: In the current era of more aggressive therapy, there has been a steady decline in the need for orthopedic surgery including joint replacements. The risk of surgically related infection or death is low, but does occur. Recent studies have shown that patients with RA undergoing arthroplasty have a low short-term (30 day) mortality risk (same as patients with osteoarthritis; odds ratio, 0.94; 0.38–2.33). Yet RA was associated with a significantly higher long-term mortality from years 1 to 8 after surgery (hazard ratio, 1.22; 1.00–1.49).[5]

EARLY RHEUMATOID ARTHRITIS

As there is no standard definition of early RA, it is best defined as "the earlier, the better." While the diagnosis of RA can be suspected with as little as 2 to 4 weeks of joint pain, 6 weeks of demonstrable synovitis in multiple joints confirms the "chronicity" required for a confident RA diagnosis (if alternative causes of chronic arthritis are excluded). Early RA clearly begins years to months before it becomes manifest polyarthritis and this is known as "preclinical RA."

Preclinical RA, by definition, includes patients who do not meet criteria for RA, but manifest arthralgia (without synovitis), are seropositive, and have a first-degree relative who has RA. A high percentage of these individuals develop increasing joint pain and swelling in the ensuing months to years, particularly in those who are anti–citrullinated protein antibody (ACPA) positive.[6]

Early presentation of inflammatory polyarthritis may also be labeled undifferentiated (inflammatory) polyarthritis or seronegative RA. Both have negative tests for RA but demonstrate the same inflammatory additive polyarthritis as RA. The difference lies with the potential to spontaneously remit. It is estimated that more than half of all patients with early inflammatory polyarthritis have undifferentiated polyarthritis (not meeting diagnostic criteria) that will go into remission within 3 to 12 months. Those that persist, and are seronegative, are labeled as seronegative RA.

In primary care, new-onset RA is less common than low back pain, osteoarthritis, gout, fibromyalgia, or psoriasis, but is more common than polymyalgia rheumatica (PMR), systemic lupus, or septic arthritis.

In 1994, there were nearly 170,000 new cases of RA in the United States. Population-based incidence rates for early RA range between 5 and 45 cases per 100,000 patients per year (patient-years).[7] Applying a conservative North American incidence rate of 20 cases per 100,000 patient-years, one might anticipate nearly 75,000 new patients with RA in the United States and 7500 in Canada in the next 12 months. This number may be doubled or more by patients who are seronegative, not meeting diagnostic criteria, or having undifferentiated inflammatory polyarthritis.

ONSET OF RHEUMATOID ARTHRITIS

Onset of RA peaks between 40 and 50 years, but is well described in all ages, including children and adolescents. Moreover, the risk of RA increases considerably after the age of 60 years. Women are affected nearly three times more often than men, but gender differences are less pronounced in older patients.

Certain populations are at greater risk of RA. The Centers for Disease Control and Prevention notes the following to be risk factors for developing RA[8]:

- Age: RA prevalence increases with age.
- Sex: RA is typically three times higher in women than men.
- Genetics: Those with the "shared epitope" have genes conferring a higher risk of developing RA and more severe RA. These genes include HLA class II genotypes (eg, HLA-DR4 or HLA-DR β1 alleles) that become relevant when exposed to environmental triggers, such as smoking or obesity. Nevertheless, these genes are not generally tested for.
- Smoking: Multiple studies show that cigarette smoking increases a person's risk of developing RA and can make the disease worse.
- Obesity: Multiple studies show obesity to be a risk factor for RA onset and also a risk factor for being refractory to standard therapies.
- Being nulliparous: Women who have never given birth may be at greater risk of developing RA.

In about two-thirds of patients, RA has an insidious onset of a symmetric additive polyarthritis. Although constitutional features (ie, malaise, fatigue, low-grade fever) may occur, it is the joint symptoms (pain, swelling, prolonged stiffness) that dominate the clinical picture. Small, medium, and large joints are equally affected. Certain features should argue against RA as a diagnosis, including an acute arthritis onset, monoarthritis, prominent weight loss, rash, or involvement of other organ systems (eg, ocular, neurologic, gastrointestinal).

DIAGNOSTIC INVESTIGATIONS

Routine laboratory studies may help in confirming the diagnosis and establishing the presence of inflammation, autoantibodies, and the risk for damage or erosions.

Acute Phase Reactants

The erythrocyte sedimentation rate (ESR) and C-reactive protein (CRP) provide surrogate evidence of inflammation. However, these may be elevated with infection; other rheumatologic disorders; malignancy; pregnancy; and chronic renal, liver, or lung disease. Moreover, in active RA, the ESR or CRP may be elevated only in 60% of patients. Thus, when elevated, these biomarkers may support an RA diagnosis, but their predictive value (positive and negative) is limited. Other laboratory studies may also indicate chronic inflammation, including an anemia of chronic disease; thrombocytosis; hypoalbuminemia; hypergammaglobulinemia; or elevated levels of ferritin, haptoglobin, or complement.

Serologic Tests

Autoantibodies have been used to guide the diagnosis of various autoimmune diseases. Testing for serologic markers may tilt the diagnostic probabilities or add prognostic value to the evaluation of inflammatory polyarthritis. The presence of RF and antinuclear antibodies is nonspecific and is found in patients with infection, malignancy, and rheumatologic diseases. These autoantibodies are present in other diseases, including viral hepatitis, systemic lupus erythematosus, cryoglobulinemia, Sjögrens syndrome, paraproteinemias, bacterial endocarditis, mycobacterial diseases, syphilis, leprosy, chronic interstitial lung disease, parasitic infections, and malignancies.

Serum rheumatoid factor (RF) is closely associated with RA and may confirm a clinically suspected diagnosis or characterize the severity of disease. RF is usually measured as an IgM antibody that binds to the Fc part of IgG. RF is found in up to 80% of established patients with RA, but may only be found in 50% of patients in the first 6 months of symptoms. RF is not specific to RA, because it is seen in 5% of the general population and up to 15% of elderly persons. RF is also positive in numerous other conditions including Sjögren syndrome, cryoglobulinemia, systemic lupus erythematosus, sarcoidosis, Waldenstrom macroglobulinemia, bacterial endocarditis, mycobacterial disease, hepatitis, chronic liver disease, leprosy, syphilis, parasitic diseases (eg, leishmaniasis), chronic interstitial lung disease, and lymphoproliferative malignancies. RF (and cyclic citrullinated peptides [CCP]/ACPA) should not be used as a screening tool, but should be ordered intelligently, in the setting of undiagnosed poly arthritis with swollen joints. Although it is true that higher titers RF (>100 IU/mL) are more likely to be RA, RF levels do not correlate with disease activity. High titers are associated with more severe RA and risk for extra-articular manifestations.[9] Lastly, other than the first 6 months, repeated or serial measurement of RF levels is rarely indicated or helpful.

Antibodies against CCP (also called ACPA) have also proven to be a useful diagnostic and staging tool, especially in early patients with RA. ACPA are nearly as sensitive as serum RF (70% CCP+ in RA of <2 years duration); But CCP antibodies are far more specific for RA (>90%+).[10] For example, although RF is often found with hepatitis C infection, ACPA is usually absent.

The presence of ACPA has been correlated with early RA, aggressive RA, radiographic damage, and shared epitope (genotype associated with RA). Moreover patients with high titers of ACPA (>250 IU/mL) or those who are double positive for RF and ACPA have a poorer prognosis.

CINCHING THE DIAGNOSIS OF RHEUMATOID ARTHRITIS

An early diagnosis requires access to medical and diagnostic services, suspicion based on onset features, and judicious use of serologic testing. RA is a clinical, and not a laboratory diagnosis. RA should be considered in the following scenarios:

- Pain, swelling, and stiffness in multiple joints going on for 12 weeks or more

- First-degree relative of a patient with RA with chronic joint symptoms (but not the lower spine or distal interphalangeal [DIP] joints)
- New-onset carpal tunnel syndrome with wrist swelling and inflammation
- Those with chronic, additive, symmetric polyarthritis affecting the proximal interphalangeal (PIP), metacarpophalangeal, wrist, and metatarsophalangeal joints
- Those meeting criteria for the diagnosis

Requisite features begin with joint pain and stiffness that improve with activity. Hallmark findings include joint swelling or effusion, and possibly warmth or erythema. **Table 1** lists the 2010 American College of Rheumatology/European League Against Rheumatism classification criteria for the diagnosis of RA.[11] Inherent to these criteria are inflammatory features and serologies that allow for an earlier diagnosis. This contrasts older criteria that relied heavily on long-standing, established disease features, such as chronicity, rheumatoid nodules, and radiographic erosions. The 2010 American College of Rheumatology/European League Against Rheumatism criteria are weighted in favor of more joints, higher titers of RF and ACPA (or CCP antibodies); and less so for acute phase reactants (ESR or CRP), duration, and large joints only. Six points or more one necesiary to diagnose RA.

DIFFERENTIAL DIAGNOSIS: OTHER CONSIDERATIONS

When patients fail to meet criteria or have atypical features, other diagnostic considerations should be considered (**Box 1**). Early RA is often confused with other

Table 1
2010 American College of Rheumatology/European League Against Rheumatism classification criteria for RA

Joint Distribution	Score
1 large joint	0
2–10 large joints	1
1–3 small joints (large joints excluded)	2
4–10 small joints (large joints excluded)	3
>10 joints (at least 1 small joint)	5
Serology	
Negative RF and negative ACPA	0
Low positive RF or ACPA ($\leq$3 × ULN)	2
High positive RF or ACPA (>3 × ULN)	3
Symptom duration	
<6 wk	0
$\geq$6 wk	1
Acute-phase reactants	
Normal CRP and ESR	0
Abnormal CRP or ESR	1

To be considered, the patient must: (1) have at least 1 joint with definite clinical synovitis (swelling), and (2) synovitis not better explained by another disease.
A score of $\geq$6 is required to have RA.
Adapted from Aletaha D, Neogi T, Silman AJ, et al. 2010 Rheumatoid arthritis classification criteria: An American College of Rheumatology/European League Against Rheumatism collaborative initiative. Arthritis Rheum 2010;62(9):2574; with permission.

Box 1
Differential diagnosis of early rheumatoid arthritis

Infection-related
  Reactive arthritis
  Viral arthritis
    Parvovirus B19
    Hepatitis B
    Hepatitis C
    Alpha viruses: chikungunya or Zika virus (mosquito-borne)

Elder onset
  Calcium pyrophosphate deposition disease rheumatoid-like arthritis
  Polymyalgia rheumatica
  Inflammatory osteoarthritis

Rheumatoid-related
  Seronegative RA
  Palindromic rheumatism
  Undifferentiated inflammatory polyarthritis
  Adult-onset Still disease, systemic lupus erythematosus

Spondylarthritis-related
  Psoriatic arthritis
  Enteropathic arthritis

---

conditions that are typically polyarticular, especially infection-related arthritides, such as reactive arthritis or viral arthritis caused by parvovirus B19, hepatitis B, hepatitis C, chikungunya virus, or Zika virus.[12] Other considerations are discussed below.

Polymyalgia Rheumatica

In the elderly (>60 years), early RA may be confused with calcium pyrophosphate deposition disease (CPPD), inflammatory osteoarthritis, and PMR. Although RA and PMR have prolonged morning stiffness, high acute phase reactants, and joint pains, PMR is distinguished from RA with prominence of limb girdle (shoulders, hips) myalgic stiffness or soreness and a lack of RF or ACPA antibodies. Yet there are patients with PMR that may resemble RA with synovitis and swelling of the hands or wrists.

Calcium Pyrophosphate Deposition Disease

CPPD and chondrocalcinosis are common in the elderly. CPPD may manifest as pseudogout attacks (involving the knee, wrist, or feet) or as chondrocalcinosis with osteoarthritis accompanied by calcification of cartilage and occasionally as chronic, somewhat inflammatory symmetric polyarthritis that resembles RA. CPPD is confirmed by arthrocentesis, identification of calcium pyrophosphate crystals, radiographic chondrocalcinosis, and negative serologic tests for RF or ACPA, although elderly patients often have a positive RF.

Inflammatory Osteoarthritis

Osteoarthritis and seropositivity increases with age. Coincident seropositivity in the presence of DIP and PIP osteoarthritic changes (Heberden and Bouchard nodes) is not uncommon, but is still just osteoarthritis with a positive RF or ACPA such is an example of the limited value of RF or ACPA in establishing a diagnosis of RA, especially at low titers. Nonetheless a minority of osteoarthritis manifests inflammatory osteoarthritis, distinguished by having inflammatory synovitis and erosive changes in multiple PIP and DIP joints of the hands. Such patients are usually seronegative and the radiograph erosions of inflammatory OA are distinctly different ("gullwing" central erosions) from that seen in RA.

Other Autoimmune Conditions

Uncommonly, other autoimmune disorders (eg, lupus, polymyositis, scleroderma) may have a polyarticular onset. Time and disease evolution will distinguish these from RA.

Spondylarthritis

Psoriatic arthritis and inflammatory bowel disease (enteropathic) arthritis may present as either an asymmetric, oligoarticular (three joints or fewer) chronic arthritis or with RA-like symmetric polyarthritis. Aside from their diagnosis affirming skin (psoriasis) or gut (Crohn) disease, they may have associated features of dactylitis, enthesitis (eg, heel pain), or sacroiliitis or spondylitis, that sets them apart from RA.

Undifferentiated polyarthritis

Studies from early arthritis clinics have shown that most new-onset, inflammatory oligoarthritis or polyarthritis will not meet criteria for the diagnosis of RA. Yet their joint involvement may have an RA-like distribution, and are distinguished from early RA by being seronegative and often go will into remission. This subset is more prevalent than early RA, and only a minority ($\leq$20%) of these patients with undifferentiated polyarthritis progress to RA. These patients are often labeled as having inflammatory arthritis, undifferentiated polyarthritis, or mistakenly as early RA. Regardless of diagnostic label, treatment of early RA and undifferentiated polyarthritis should match the degree and duration of synovitis and not be dictated by the diagnostic criteria.

Palindromic rheumatism

Palindromic rheumatism is an uncommon disorder linked to RA because occasionally patients with RA initially present with a palindromic pattern. It is characterized by recurrent, afebrile attacks of monoarthritis or tendonitis, occasionally polyarthritis, usually lasting hours to days. Pain, swelling, and redness occur in typical RA joints (eg, wrists, shoulders, ankles, knees, metatarsophalangeal, and fingers). Less than half of patients are seropositive and seropositivity increases the odds of evolving into chronic RA. Nearly half of affected patients experience chronic, intermittent palindromic attacks; in 30% to 40% the condition evolves into RA; and up to 15% go into clinical remission. Palindromic rheumatism needs to be distinguished from early RA, and other recurrent arthropathies, such as crystalline arthritis, Behçet disease, or familial Mediterranean fever. Patients with recurrent attacks may benefit from intra-articular or oral corticosteroids, antimalarial drugs, or disease-modifying antirheumatic drug (DMARD) therapy.

Adult-onset Still disease

Still disease is a variant of juvenile idiopathic arthritis (previously called juvenile RA). Adult-onset Still disease is a febrile inflammatory disorder of young adults with hallmark features of quotidian fevers, evanescent rashes, and polyarthritis.[13] Although polyarthritis is seen in up to 80% of patients with adult-onset Still disease, nearly 30% develop an erosive, RA-like arthritis that often requires treatment with DMARDs or biologics.

NOT RHEUMATOID ARTHRITIS!

There are several scenarios that should not be confused with early RA, but often are, usually because of overinterpretation of polyarthralgias and rheumatoid serologies.

Critical to the RA diagnosis is the objective finding of swollen, inflamed joints. It should be noted that RA is not:

- Induced by trauma.
- Caused or cured by diet alone.
- Arthralgia (joint pain): one needs to demonstrate synovitis or swollen joints to consider RA.
- Hand deformity: hand deformities do occur in RA, but also osteoarthritis, psoriatic arthritis, gout, and other autoimmune diseases.
- Low back or DIP joint arthritis.
- Widespread pain with fatigue: such patients are more likely to have fibromyalgia.
- Lyme disease: RA should not be confused with Lyme arthritis. The latter only occurs in those who live in or travel to Lyme disease–endemic areas and who usually had demonstrated the bulls-eye rash called erythema chronicum migrans. Serologic testing for Lyme disease is far less predictive than these clinical requirements for the diagnosis. Lyme arthritis is a late manifestation of Lyme disease and usually presents as intermittent or persistent inflammatory arthritis in a few large joints, especially the knee, shoulder, ankle, elbow, or wrist. It does not appear as a chronic, additive, symmetric polyarthritis of large and small joints, typical of RA.

RULES FOR REFERRAL

Once the diagnosis of RA is suspected or confirmed, the primary care or diagnosing physician should develop a treatment plan, initiate therapy, and consider referral. The goal is to reduce the time from symptom onset to diagnosis, and to reduce the time from diagnosis to the initiation DMARD therapy.

Early referral is necessary as MRI studies have shown articular erosions are seen as early as 12 to 16 weeks from the onset. Within the first 3 years, nearly 70% of patients have radiographic damage. These data underscore the need for prompt diagnosis, treatment, and referral. Referral is necessary to confirm the RA diagnosis and initiate prompt DMARD therapy. A recent UK National Health Service study of 822 patients with RA showed the median time between symptom onset and rheumatology consult was 27.2 weeks and that only 20% of patients were seen within the first 3 months of symptom onset.[14]

Ideally, all patients with recent-onset RA or inflammatory arthritis should be evaluated by a rheumatologist. Diagnostic certainty may be fleeting in early disease because the symptoms are not fully developed, seropositivity is lower in the first 6 months, and outcomes of new-onset polyarthritis vary.[15]

Emery and colleagues[16] have developed rules for early arthritis referral to a rheumatologist:

1. Three or more swollen joints
2. A positive metacarpophalangeal or metatarsophalangeal squeeze test to elicit pain
3. Morning stiffness of 30 minutes or more in relevant joints
4. Joint symptoms of greater than 6 weeks but less than 6 months
5. An abnormal serologic test (RF, CCP) or elevated ESR or CRP

TREATMENT CHOICES IN EARLY RHEUMATOID ARTHRITIS

It is the clinician's task to address the patient's pain, swelling, and stiffness with effective interventions. There are three modalities that every clinician should address in early RA: (1) analgesics, (2) corticosteroids, and (3) DMARDs.

Analgesics

The initial goal is to minimize pain, inflammation, and functional impairment. Analgesic therapy, splinting, and physical therapy should be liberally prescribed soon after onset and used until a diagnosis is established. Analgesic agents include acetaminophen, tramadol, nonacetylated salicylates, nonsteroidal anti-inflammatory drugs, or low-dose prednisone. These can be used at the lowest effective dose. For instance, a patient with new-onset RA with swollen PIPs and knees could be given any of the following (noting limits imposed by comorbidities and contraindications):

- Extended-release acetaminophen, 650 mg, two tablets twice daily
- Meloxicam, 7.5 mg daily or twice daily (with meals)
- Tramadol, 50 mg twice or three times daily as needed
- Prednisone, 5 mg daily

Pain is a prevalent feature in early RA and is most often related to inflammation, rather than damage. Thus, strong narcotic or addictive analgesics should be avoided and prohibited in patients with early RA.

Corticosteroids

Patients with slowly progressive or aggressive RA may achieve short-term benefits from injectable or low-dose oral corticosteroids while waiting for DMARD therapies (MTX, hydroxychloroquine [HCQ], or sulfasalazine [SSZ]) to be in effect. It is paramount to note that steroids are acutely wonderful and chronically dangerous. Even low doses of prednisone (5 mg per day) carry a significantly increased risk of serious or hospitalizeable infections, and higher rated of CV events and comorbidities (diabetes, osteoporosis) with doses greater than 5 mg daily. Dosing steroids in early RA should be at the lowest dose effective and possible (2.5 mg is preferred over 5 mg or 7.5 mg daily) and only until DMARD or biologic therapies have controlled the synovitis. Hence, most patients only need to be on low-dose oral corticosteroids for less than 4 months. Lastly, intra-articular corticosteroids usually used in the knee and shoulder can provide effective short-term relief in those patients with disproportionate symptoms from one or a few joints.

Disease-Modifying Therapy

DMARDs include conventional synthetic DMARDs (eg, MTX, HCQ, SSZ, and leflunomide) and biologic DMARDs (eg, etanercept, adalimumab, abatacept, and tocilizumab). Currently there are numerous Food and Drug Administration approved DMARDs for use in RA: 6 conventional DMARDs (eg, MTX, SSZ, HCQ), 9 biologic DMARDs, and 13 biosimilar DMARDs (copies of etanercept, adalimumab, infliximab, or rituximab).

The primary care physician should start conventional DMARD therapy soon after the diagnosis, with either HCQ or MTX, while referring the patient to the rheumatologist for ongoing DMARD management. HCQ tends to have far less side effects than MTX, but does not have the overall efficacy of MTX. Starting doses for these agents are:

- HCQ, 200 mg: one or two tablets per day (dosed as 4–5 mg/kg/d)
- MTX, 2.5 mg: four tablets given once a week (eg, every Friday) along with daily folic acid, 2 mg per day

Patients taking HCQ require little monitoring but do need a baseline eye examination soon after starting HCQ therapy. Patients taking MTX should be tested for hepatitis before use and have laboratory studies at 1 month and 3 months after starting and then every 3 months to monitor for cytopenia or hepatotoxicity.

With referral, to the rheumatologist confirms the diagnosis; fine tunes the use of analgesics, steroids, and DMARD therapy; and involves adjunctive providers (physical therapy, orthopedists) when needed. Moreover, rheumatologic services can further advise the patient on numerous issues including lifestyle issues (weight loss, smoking cessation), future pregnancies, vaccination safety CV risks associated with RA, work and ergonomic adjustments, and future prognosis.

CONSEQUENCES OF DELAYED INTERVENTION

Numerous studies have demonstrated the advantage of early and aggressive treatment, even with older DMARDs, such as gold and HCQ.[17] Numerous treatment options exist for patients with early RA. Early institution of appropriately aggressive treatment can dramatically improve the patient's synovitis, quality of life, and lessen joint destruction and the future need for hospitalization and orthopedic surgery. Thus, there is a critical window of opportunity to diagnose and treat early RA as soon as possible.[18] Early recognition, diagnosis, DMARD initiation, and partnering with a rheumatologist is a proven formula, wherein, patients captured in the first 3 to 12 months of their disease can manage their disease and optimize long-term outcomes.

CLINICS CARE POINTS

- RA is not a laboratory diagnosis; up to 20% of patients are seronegative.
- Polyarthritis lasting more than 6 weeks is required.
- An additive, symmetric polyarthritis of small and large joints is evident at disease onset.
- Do not wait for classic features (nodules, erosions, deformity) because they are seen late.
- Only use corticosteroids as bridge therapy while waiting for DMARDs to be effective.
- Start DMARD therapy and refer as soon as the diagnosis is made.

DISCLOSURE

None.

REFERENCES

1. Cush JJ, Weinblatt ME, Kavanaugh A. In: Weinblatt ME, Kavanaugh A, editors. Rheumatoid arthritis. J. J. Cush. 4th edition. New York (NY): Professional Communications; 2014.
2. Turesson C. Comorbidity in rheumatoid arthritis. Swiss Med Wkly 2016;146: w14290.
3. Bongartz T, Nannini C, Medina-Velasquez YF, et al. Incidence and mortality of interstitial lung disease in rheumatoid arthritis: a population-based study. Arthritis Rheum 2010;62(6):1583–91.
4. Sparks JA, Chang SC, Liau KP, et al. Rheumatoid Arthritis and Mortality Among Women During 36 Years of Prospective Follow-Up: Results From the Nurses Health Study. Arthritis Care Res 2016;68(6):753–62.

5. Michaud K, Fehringer EV, Garvin K, et al. Rheumatoid arthritis patients are not at increased risk for 30-day cardiovascular events, infections, or mortality after total joint arthroplasty. Arthritis Res Ther 2013;15(6):R195.
6. Tracy A, Buckley CD, Raza K. Pre-symptomatic autoimmunity in rheumatoid arthritis: when does the disease start? Semin Immunopathol 2017;39:423–35.
7. Alarcon GS. Epidemiology of rheumatoid arthritis. Rheum Dis Clin North Am 1995;21:589–604.
8. Centers for Disease Control and Prevention. What are the risk factors for RA?. Available at: https://www.cdc.gov/arthritis/basics/rheumatoid-arthritis.html. Accessed October 25, 2020.
9. Nielsen SF, Bojesen SE, Schnohr P, et al. Elevated rheumatoid factor and long term risk of rheumatoid arthritis: a prospective cohort study. BMJ 2012;345: e5244.
10. Kroot EJ, de Jong BA, van Leeuwen MA, et al. The prognostic value of anti-cyclic citrullinated peptide antibody in patients with recent-onset rheumatoid arthritis. Arthritis Rheum 2000;43(8):1831–5.
11. Aletaha D, Neogi T, Silman AJ, et al. 2010 Rheumatoid arthritis classification criteria: an American College of Rheumatology/European League Against Rheumatism collaborative initiative. Arthritis Rheum 2010;62:2569.
12. Cush JJ. Mosquito arthritis. RheumNow.com;2016. Available at: https:// rheumnow.com/content/mosquito-arthritis. Accessed October 25, 2020.
13. Cush JJ. Adult onset Still's disease. Bull Rheum Dis 2000;49(6):1–4.
14. Stack RJ, Nightingale P, Jinks C, et al. Delays between the onset of symptoms and first rheumatology consultation in patients with rheumatoid arthritis in the UK: an observational study. BMJ Open 2019;9(3):e024361.
15. Cush JJ. Criteria for early referrals from primary care. RheumNow.com: August 9, 2017. Available at: https://rheumnow.com/content/criteria-early-referrals-primary-care. Accessed October 25, 2020.
16. Emery P, Breedveld FC, Dougados M, et al. Early referral recommendation for newly diagnosed rheumatoid arthritis: evidence based development of a clinical guide. Ann Rheum Dis 2002;61(4):290–7.
17. Tsakonas E, Fitzgerald AA, Fitzcharles MA, et al. Consequences of delayed therapy with second-line agents in rheumatoid arthritis: a 3 year followup on the hydroxychloroquine in early rheumatoid arthritis (HERA) study. J Rheumatol 2000; 27(3):623–9.
18. Cush JJ. Early rheumatoid arthritis: is there a window of opportunity? J Rheumatol Suppl 2007;80:1–7.

Management of Knee Osteoarthritis
What Internists Need to Know

Joel A. Block, MD*, Dmitriy Cherny, MD

KEYWORDS

- Osteoarthritis • Knee pain • Nerve growth factor • Placebo effect
- Platelet rich plasma

KEY POINTS

- Osteoarthritis (OA) is a clinical diagnosis, not a radiographic or laboratory diagnosis; as structural degeneration accompanies normal aging, clinical OA is defined by the presence of pain.
- As there is no therapy that alters the natural history of OA in people, therapy is focused on palliation of pain and retention of function.
- Therapy should include nonpharmacologic interventions such as self-efficacy, weight loss when appropriate, and exercise, preferably with the involvement of physical therapy.
- When pharmacotherapy is necessary to manage pain, nonsteroidal anti-inflammatory drugs (NSAIDs) remain the mainstay of therapy when not contraindicated. Both topical and oral NSAIDs may be used. Intra-articular interventions, such as glucocorticoids, may be effective for short-term pain relief.
- OA pain is sensitive to the placebo effect. Widely marketed interventions, such as intraarticular stem cell therapy and platelet-rich plasma, are expensive and have not been demonstrated to be superior to the prominent placebo effect for knee OA pain.

Among musculoskeletal diseases, osteoarthritis (OA) is by far the most common form of arthritis and results in vast morbidity and societal costs. It is estimated that the overall costs to society represent more than 0.5% of the gross domestic product of industrialized countries[1]; in the United States, OA accounts for almost $200 billion annually in medical costs,[2] and symptomatically, it affects more than 25 million Americans, approximately 10% of the adult population.[2,3] Moreover, adults are estimated to have a 40% to 50% lifetime risk of developing clinically significant OA.[4] The dramatic advances in therapeutics for inflammatory arthritis in recent years have not been

This article originally appeared in the Medical Clinics of North America, Volume 105, Issue 2, March 2021.
Division of Rheumatology, Rush University Medical Center, 1611 West Harrison Street, Suite 510, Chicago, IL 60612, USA
* Corresponding author.
E-mail address: jblock@rush.edu

matched by comparable progress in OA. Hence, OA patients seen in routine Rheumatology care today have significantly worse clinical status than those with rheumatoid arthritis (RA),[5] and can expect to derive substantially less improvement with modern care.[6] However, careful examination of the status of patients with OA and RA revealed that even prior to the advent of the biologic therapies, those with OA had comparable pain and functional disability to those with RA.[7] Although OA can affect any diarthrodial joint, certain areas are more predisposed than others, and OA of the knees is among the most common and most debilitating sites. This article provides a narrative, evidence-based review of current management of OA of the knees, with emphasis on topical and injectable therapies.

DEFINITION

Historically, OA was considered a disease of degenerative cartilage, and hence therapeutic strategies throughout most of the 20th century were devoted to protecting and repairing articular cartilage. Fundamentally, however, that perspective failed to account for the widespread changes that occur throughout all joint tissues. In addition, as cartilage is not innervated, the source of OA-related pain in a cartilage-centric paradigm remained a mystery. It is now clear that OA is a degenerative process that involves all joint tissues, and therefore, to be effective, therapeutic strategies must deal with the entire joint. In addition, pain is now appreciated to be fundamental to the clinical condition of OA, and whereas structural degeneration of joints is a universal feature of normal aging, the disease of OA is not. By late middle age, virtually everyone has evidence of cartilage degeneration,[8] but clinical OA is present in only a minority of people, even among those with evidence of structural joint degeneration.[9] Although for large-scale epidemiologic studies, structural joint changes evident by radiography have been used to define the presence of OA, there is substantial discordance between radiographic OA and actual disease. Hence, a reasonable definition of OA is: "a joint disease that consists of painful degeneration affecting all joint tissues, and involves progressive deterioration of articular cartilage and alterations of subchondral bone and surrounding joint structures; local inflammation may be present but is not the primary source of joint dysfunction."[10]

CLINICAL PRESENTATION

The cardinal manifestation of knee OA is pain. Structural degeneration in a joint accompanies normal aging, is often asymptomatic, and may precede the development of clinical symptoms by years or decades. OA manifests as disease when the patient notices pain or dysfunction. OA pain is generally first noticed during loading of the involved joint; hence with knee OA, early symptoms occur while standing or walking. With disease progression, pain may become persistent even at rest. Knee pain may wax and wane during the disease course, and it is typical to have prolonged pain-free periods punctuated by painful flares that may last weeks or months. Other symptoms of knee OA include subjective joint instability and the gelling phenomenon, wherein the joint feels stiff transiently as the patient stands. Additionally, patients may notice decreased range of motion of the knee, and as the knees are superficial, they may notice prominent bony bumps cosmetically, which are caused by osteophytes. Physical examination of the OA knee often reveals crepitance, and frequently a cool effusion may be detected. It is important to note that the diagnosis of OA is a clinical diagnosis; there are no laboratory tests that are abnormal because of OA. Radiographically, the OA joint may have osteophytes, asymmetric joint space narrowing, subchondral sclerosis, and occasionally subchondral cysts. Nonetheless, radiographic abnormalities alone may be asymptomatic and thus do not imply clinical OA.[11] Moreover, the focus of therapy ought to be directed at symptom palliation and retention of function rather than structural degeneration. This is especially important with regards to the decision to proceed with surgical intervention for OA, which should be made strictly on the basis of clinical severity and not determined by the radiographic severity of OA. It is important to distinguish OA from the inflammatory arthritides, which are discussed in the rest of this issue. Rather than presenting with systemic symptoms, OA is not associated with diffuse synovitis or symptoms characteristic of systemic inflammatory disease (**Table 1**). Whereas patients with inflammatory arthritis such as RA experience prolonged stiffness in the morning, OA specifically presents with no or transient stiffness, such as the brief gelling phenomenon felt after a period of inactivity. In addition, OA joints tend to have palpable bony enlargements (osteophytes) and are either not inflamed or have a mild inflammatory response, with less than 2000 leukocytes/μL upon arthrocentesis. Meanwhile, rheumatoid joints are highly inflamed, erythematous, with boggy synovium, and effusions with greater than 2000 leukocytes/μL. It is equally important to distinguish OA from common extra-articular sources of knee pain, such as anserine bursitis, which presents as significant medial knee pain exacerbated by climbing stairs or rising from a chair; this is diagnosed by point tenderness over the anserine bursa at the proximal medial tibia. Although anserine bursitis may accompany knee OA, it is distinguished from OA pain by its focal localization which is extra-articular and sensitive to palpation.

APPROACH TO THERAPY

To date, there are no therapies that have been shown to alter the natural history of OA in people. The prevention of structural progression remains purely aspirational. Hence, the main goals of contemporary OA therapy are to palliate pain and to retain function. Recently, the American College of Rheumatology (ACR) and the Osteoarthritis Research Society International (OARSI) have published updated guidelines for the nonoperative management of knee OA.[12,13] These are largely concordant, and stress both nonpharmacological and pharmacologic modalities (**Table 2**).

NONPHARMACOLOGICAL APPROACHES TO OSTEOARTHRITIS

There is consensus that patients benefit from education and programs aimed at self-efficacy and self-management techniques, as part of a holistic approach to knee OA. These help patients to set realistic expectations and have been shown to be beneficial to patients' quality of life.[14] As knee OA is a chronic lifelong condition, and most patients become mildly symptomatic years before they develop severe daily pain, it is important for physicians to educate all such patients about the importance of noninvasive physical measures. Most will benefit from physical therapy, where they are taught exercise regimens, and undergo supervised range-of-motion and functional training. Additional adjunctive relief can be obtained by icing painful joints, especially before and after activity; some people prefer local heat to ice.

Weight Loss

Obesity is a significant risk factor both for incident knee OA and for progression of disease. Although sustained weight loss is impractical for a large number of patients, there is evidence that those who are able to lose weight derive substantial clinical benefit.[15] There appears to be a dose response between the magnitude of clinical benefit and the amount of sustained weight loss in knee OA, such that significant

Table 1
The typical clinical features of osteoarthritis compared and contrasted with those of the inflammatory arthritides

	Osteoarthritis	Inflammatory Arthritides
History	• Worse with prolonged use or loading • Morning stiffness <30 min • Gelling phenomenon • Subjective joint instability	• Often improved with prolonged use • Morning stiffness >30 min
Physical examination	• Cool effusion • Varus/valgus deformity • Bony hypertrophy • Crepitance with damage	• Warm effusion • Skin erythema • Boggy swelling • Significant tenderness to palpation • Crepitance with damage
Laboratory findings	• No specific abnormalities	• Elevated ESR/CRP • Hypoalbuminemia • Anemia of chronic disease • Thrombocytosis • Positive autoimmune serologies
Synovial fluid	• <2000 leukocytes/µL, lymphocytic predominance • Incident CPPD crystals possible	• 2000- >50,000 leukocytes/µL, neutrophil predominance
Imaging	• Asymmetric joint space narrowing • Subchondral sclerosis and cysts • Osteophytosis • Meniscal or ligamentous damage with progression	• Dependent on subtype

The diagnosis of OA is a clinical decision not dependent on laboratory or radiographic features, and OA is distinct from the inflammatory arthritides, as it is not associated with systemic symptoms or with systemic inflammation.

Table 2
A summary of the recently updated treatment guidelines for knee osteoarthritis, as published by the Osteoarthritis Research Society International and by the American College of Rheumatology

Treatment Modality	OARSI	ACR
Nonpharmacological		
Exercise	Yes, for all patients	Yes, for all patients
Physical therapy	Yes, for all patients	Yes, for all patients
Eastern disciplines (yoga, tai chi)	Yes, for all patients, preference for tai chi	Yes, for all patients, preference for tai chi
Weight reduction, if overweight	Yes, for all patients	Yes, for all patients
Self-management and education	Yes, for all patients	Yes, for all patients
Biomechanical (cane)	Recommended	Recommended
Unloading knee braces	Not recommended	Recommended
Heat/therapeutic cooling	Conditionally recommended	Conditionally recommended
Balance training	Conditionally recommended	Conditionally recommended
Cognitive behavioral therapy	Conditionally recommended	Conditionally recommended
Pharmacologic		
Topical NSAIDs	Strongly recommended	Strongly recommended
Topical capsaicin	Not recommended	Conditionally recommended
Acetaminophen	Conditionally not recommended	Conditionally recommended: short-term use
Tramadol	Uncertain	Conditionally recommended
Oral NSAIDs or COX-2 inhibitors	Conditionally recommended	Strongly recommended when not medically contraindicated
Duloxetine	In appropriate circumstances	In appropriate circumstances
Opiates	Not recommended	Conditionally not recommended
Intra-articular glucocorticoids	Conditionally recommended	Recommended
Intra-articular hyaluronans	Conditionally recommended	Conditionally not recommended
PRP	Strongly recommended against	Strongly recommended against
Mesenchymal stem cell therapy	Strongly recommended against	Strongly recommended against
Anti-NGF therapy	Not addressed	Not addressed
Complementary		

(continued on next page)

Table 2 (continued)		
Treatment Modality	**OARSI**	**ACR**
Acupuncture	Uncertain	In appropriate circumstances
Glucosamine and/or chondroitin sulfate	Strongly recommended against	Strongly recommended against
TENS	Strongly recommended against	Strongly recommended against
Therapeutic Ultrasonography	No recommendation	Conditionally recommended
Kinesiotaping	Not recommended	Conditionally recommended

Abbreviations: COX-2, cytotoxygenase-2; OARSI, osteoarthritis research society international; TENS, transcutaneous electrical nerve stimulation.
aThis table summarizes the major recommendations of each organization shown and is not intended to represent a complete listing of their guidelines. There is overall concordance regarding recommendations, although some variation exists.
Adapted from Kolasinski SL, Neogi T, Hochberg MC, et al. 2019 American College of Rheumatology/Arthritis Foundation Guideline for the Management of Osteoarthritis of the Hand, Hip, and Knee. Arthritis Rheumatol 2020;72(2):220-233; and Bannuru RR, Osani MC, Vaysbrot EE, et al. OARSI guidelines for the non-surgical management of knee, hip, and polyarticular osteoarthritis. Osteoarthritis Cartilage 2019;27(11):1578-1589; with permission.

effects are noted at a loss of 5% of body mass, and benefit increases dramatically as the amount of weight loss increases, up to at least 20% in very overweight individuals.[16]

Exercise and Muscle Strengthening

Patients who exercise regularly have reduced knee OA pain, and formal exercise training regimens supervised by physical therapists provide significant pain relief.[17,18] The original intention of such regimens for knee OA was to provide biomechanical unloading by strengthening the periarticular musculature. Although the mechanical benefit of such programs has not been borne out and there is no evidence that these programs alter structural progression, the pain advantage is unambiguous. There is insufficient evidence to support a particular modality of exercise over others[12]; rather, it appears that aerobic conditioning of all types provides pain relief. The most common exercise is walking, which should be encouraged among knee OA patients. Swimming and cycling are considered lower-impact activities, and are often preferred as the reduced loading of arthritic knees may perhaps be better tolerated. In addition, neuromuscular training and balance training are often advocated, although without a full database to support them in OA. Nonetheless, neuromuscular training may assist in reducing falls and knee injuries.[19]

In addition to standard exercise regimens, there has been attention to Eastern practices as potential adjuncts for palliating knee OA. Tai Chi is the modality that has the most supportive information in OA, and is now strongly recommended by the recent ACR[12] and OARSI[13] guidelines. Yoga is also popular, may be beneficial, and is also recommended by the updated guidelines.

Mechanical Unloading

It has been accepted for years that progression of knee OA is mediated by aberrant biomechanical loading,[20] and it has been expected that amelioration of the abnormal loading would provide salutary effects both on structural progression and on pain. Various noninvasive mechanically active strategies have been identified, which have been shown to have beneficial effects on knee loading, although none have been demonstrated to affect disease progression. Importantly, the simple use of a cane while walking can yield substantial unloading effects across the knee[21] and provides stability for patients who feel subjective knee buckling or for those who may have unsteady gait. Additional unloading can be accomplished by using bilateral walking sticks.[22] However, despite the mechanical benefits of cane use, there is no evidence that it has a beneficial structural effect on the disease.[23] Valgus unloading knee braces have been approved by the US Food and Drug Administration (FDA) for many years for the pain of medial knee OA, and they do provide mechanical benefit by reducing loads across the arthritic knee. For people who tolerate them, they may provide an important option for noninvasive care, and they are recommended by the updated ACR guidelines.[12] Thus, it may be worthwhile to try braces, generally facilitated by referral to Physical Medicine and Rehabilitation. Nonetheless, many patients find them cumbersome, unsightly, and uncomfortable, and there is insufficient evidence for their actual efficacy to expect that they will be helpful in most patients.[24]

PHARMACOLOGIC APPROACH TO OSTEOARTHRITIS

As knee OA is a chronic, progressive, lifelong disease, most patients will eventually require more than adjunctive measures to control their pain. This implies pharmacologic intervention. As there are no strategies that have been shown to delay disease progression or to modify the course of the disease over time, pharmacologic approaches focus on control of pain and maintenance of function while limiting adverse reactions.

TOPICAL THERAPIES

Topically administered medications have relatively limited systemic absorption, and have been shown to be effective for OA pain, at least in superficial joints. As many OA patients are elderly and have comorbid conditions that may preclude long-term NSAID use, a trial of topical therapy may be preferred. Some authorities recommend topical capsaicin, which is available without prescription in the United States and has been approved for use in knee OA for many years. It is thought to act by depletion of Substance P and to reduce the sensitivity of peripheral nociceptors,[25] and has been shown to have pain-palliating effects in OA if used 4 times daily. It must be applied cautiously, and the hands washed thoroughly after application, because exposure to mucous membranes causes significant burning pain, as capsaicin is the active ingredient in hot peppers. The aggregate experience, however, suggests that topical capsaicin may provide only minor pain relief in OA, and a Cochrane Collaboration systematic review, which found short-term pain advantages, concluded that only some patients will feel substantial relief long term.[26] In addition, there appear to be adverse events in 80% of the cases, for the reasons noted previously.[27]

An important option is topical NSAIDs. In the United States, diclofenac gel is now available both by prescription and over the counter; in other countries, additional NSAIDs are topical options, including ibuprofen and ketoprofen. These tend to be well tolerated and may be used in many situations where systemic NSAIDs are contraindicated. Topical salicylates have also been an option in combination preparations over the counter. Diclofenac gel has been approved by the FDA for the treatment of knee OA and has been shown to be more effective than placebo in short-term (less than 6 weeks) and longer-term (12 weeks) studies in clinical trials.[28] An over-the-counter preparation is now available without prescription.

ORAL THERAPIES

Eventually, most OA patients will require more than topical therapy to control their pain. Although various options exist, OA pain remains incompletely treated in many patients, and is widely recognized as a major unmet medical need.

Acetaminophen

For many years, acetaminophen was recommended by most societies' guidelines for the initial treatment of knee OA. This was on the basis of perceived safety and an early study suggesting equivalence to oral ibuprofen in a short 4-week trial.[29] However, when acetaminophen was tested against placebo as well as against an NSAID positive control in a 12-week trial, which is more relevant to the chronic pain of OA, it was found to lose its efficacy after 4 weeks and to be indistinguishable from placebo by 12 weeks.[30] This was eventually confirmed by multiple other trials, which suggested the lack of a clinically relevant benefit.[31] In addition, acetaminophen has been implicated in a large number of accidental cases of fulminant hepatic failure because of accidental overdose. As such, it may still be useful for short-term painful flares in OA, but ought not be used in the chronic care of OA, and it has now been removed as a recommendation by OARSI.[13]

Nonsteroidal Anti-inflammatory Drugs

As a category, nonsteroidal anti-inflammatory drugs (NSAIDs) represent the most effective and widely available oral therapy for knee OA, and they remain the mainstay of OA therapy. For analgesia, they have been shown to be superior to placebo and pure analgesics, and to retain their activity during long-term use.[32,33] There are many NSAID preparations that are available, both by prescription and over the counter, and all are largely equi-efficacious at full doses.[34] A recent network meta-analysis that had suggested some benefit of diclofenac over naproxen or ibuprofen was subsequently retracted (Lancet, DOI:https://doi.org/10.1016/S0140-6736(16)30002-2). Despite their efficacy, chronic use of NSAIDs entails some risk, especially among many patients with OA. They must be used with caution in patients with cardiac disease, renal impairment, or who are at risk of gastrointestinal (GI) bleeding. Generally, those who are middle-aged or older, or who are at increased risk of gastritis are treated concomitantly with gastric-neutralizing therapy, such as proton pump inhibitors or misoprostol; alternatively, the use of cyclooxygenase-2 inhibitors such as celecoxib may be safer for the GI tract and for patients who take anticoagulation therapy. Regular monitoring of renal function and of blood counts is important for all patients who are taking NSAIDs chronically. With such measures, however, NSAIDs may be safely used in a large number of OA patients, many of whom cannot attain similar levels of relief with other classes of therapeutics.

Neuroactive Medications

When OA was considered to be an isolated disease of degenerative cartilage, therapy was directed at ameliorating the local pain and inflammation caused by such processes. As a result, the primary strategy involved use of anti-inflammatories, such as NSAIDs and intra-articular glucocorticoids, as well as analgesics. However, it is now appreciated that OA pain has a complex pathophysiology, and in addition to the nociceptive component, which conventional analgesics target, there may also be components of inflammatory, neuropathic, and dysfunctional pain that require different strategies for relief.[35] Neuroactive agents may be helpful with both the neuropathic components and the chronic pain components of OA pain. Duloxetine, a serotonin and norepinephrine reuptake inhibitor (SNRI), has been shown to be superior to placebo for OA pain.[36] It has been approved by the FDA for use in OA and musculoskeletal pain since 2010, and it may be used to relieve the complex pain of knee OA. Other agents that are widely used to treat neuropathic pain and depression have not been formally approved for the OA indication by the FDA; nonetheless, many, such as gabapentin, pregabalin, and other selective serotonin reuptake inhibitors (SSRIs) and SNRIs, are used clinically by many physicians to treat chronic pain, including chronic OA pain.

Opioids

Opioids have long been used effectively to control acute pain; however, their role in chronic nonmalignant pain has been controversial. There is abundant evidence that opiates effectively palliate OA pain.[37] However, there is substantially less evidence that they retain efficacy over long periods, and, importantly, they are associated with greatly increased risk of adverse effects.[38] Some of these, such as falling,[39] may be life-threatening in the elderly. As a result, opioids are no longer recommended in the ACR[12] and OARSI[13] guidelines for use in OA pain, and are not widely used by OA authorities.

Tramadol is a weak opiate agonist that has been shown to have efficacy in pain modification and is approved for use in OA. Earlier data suggested that a clinically significant pain reduction would be achieved by a substantial minority of patients, although at the cost of high prevalence of adverse events, principally GI upset.[40] With greater experience and large numbers treated, it has appeared that the efficacy of tramadol may be less significant than previously reported,[41] and guidance regarding the cost-benefit analysis remains uncertain. Nevertheless, tramadol remains in widespread use clinically in the United States, as there is a paucity of alternatives to NSAIDs for refractory OA pain.

INTRA-ARTICULAR THERAPIES
Glucocorticoids

Glucocorticoids have been delivered intraarticularly for several decades to treat the pain of OA. It is widely acknowledged that they may provide short-term relief, but there remains controversy regarding the magnitude of the benefit, and the severity of associated risks. In addition, there is little evidence to suggest that the relief from such therapy is prolonged.[42] A recent clinical trial evaluated intra-articular injections of solumedrol every 3 months and reported that after 2 years, there was no benefit to pain or function over placebo injections, but there was some evidence of more rapid degradation of articular cartilage in the treated group,[43] suggesting that there may be some risk to prolonged glucocorticoid exposure of the articular cartilage, and providing evidence for the long-held belief that any joint should not be injected more than a few times each year. There does not appear to be compelling evidence that any particular form of glucocorticoid is substantially superior to the others for intra-articular use. Of interest, a novel preparation of long-acting triamcinolone (triamcinolone acetonide extended-release injectable suspension) has recently been approved for intraarticular use in OA; it may provide a pain advantage over conventional triamcinolone in the first few weeks, but appears to be equivalent by 12 weeks.[44]

Hyaluronan

Hyaluronan, formerly called hyaluronic acid (HA), is an unsulfated glycosaminoglycan that is present throughout the extracellular matrix in many tissues and has diverse functions in growth, development, and in maintaining structural integrity. In articular cartilage, it forms enormous aggregates with the large aggregating proteoglycan aggrecan; these aggregates, which have very high negative charge densities, are trapped in a collagen network and provide the mechanical stiffness that permits cartilage to cushion the bones during loading. Hyaluronan is also present in synovial fluid and augments nonboundary lubrication during articulation. Hyaluronan was originally developed therapeutically as a viscosupplement in an effort to improve joint function in OA, and to thereby retard disease progression. However, after injection, it is cleared rapidly from the joint, and any biomechanical advantage is lost within several hours. Nonetheless, it was observed that some people had significant pain relief after hyaluronan injections, and that pain relief at times was durable. On the basis of those observations, several preparations of hyaluronan have been developed and approved for use by the FDA for intra-articular use in knee OA.[45] There remains controversy regarding the magnitude of benefit above the placebo effect, and professional societies disagree on its utility. Whereas OARSI conditionally recommends its use,[13] the ACR conditionally does not recommend it.[12] Nonetheless, there is evidence that for people who obtain a salutary response from HA, the response may last for several months,[46] and when incorporating the placebo response, the total benefit (of the active agent added to the placebo response) may be substantial.[45] The cost of HA is high relative to the limited increment above placebo, the average wholesale acquisition cost being between $750 and $1400 for each dosing cycle, and hence most authorities use it sparingly.

BIOLOGIC THERAPIES

In light of the vast societal costs and morbidity resulting from knee OA, and the fact that conventional medical therapy cannot fully alleviate the pain and dysfunction caused by the disease, there is an enormous market for more effective therapeutics that would at least relieve the pain, and preferably would delay OA structural progression. As a result, the pharmaceutical industry has invested vast resources in discovery, and there is a pipeline of potential agents. Many of these targets have been revealed by new knowledge regarding the pathophysiology and neurobiology of OA pain.[47,48] Currently, there are no biologic agents that have been approved for use in OA; however, at least 1 group of monoclonal antibodies is far along in development.

Antinerve Growth Factor

The target that is most advanced in clinical trials of knee OA therapeutics is antinerve growth factor (anti-NGF). NGF was originally described by Rita Levi-Montalcini and Stanley Cohen in 1951 for its role promoting neuronal growth and survival in check embryos.[49] In the 1990s, while under investigation as a potential therapeutic for peripheral neuropathies, it was found to result in rapid-onset hyperalgesia that prevented further development, and in fact was potently pronociceptive.[47] This observation led to the development of neutralizing antibodies directed against NGF, and for trials in various painful conditions. The first large-scale phase 2 trial for knee OA was published in 2010[50] and reported substantial relief of knee OA pain. Shortly thereafter, however, the FDA imposed a halt on clinical testing in OA because of the occurrence of rapidly progressive OA, including in otherwise uninvolved joints, and a concern of avascular necrosis. After extensive testing and evaluation, the clinical hold was lifted in 2015, and trials were permitted to resume, subject to stringent mitigation strategies and lower doses. Although there are 2 antibodies that continue in clinical development, tanezumab and fasinumab, phase 3 trials have recently been published using tanezumab.[51,52] There appears to be a significant pain benefit to anti-NGF, stronger at 5.0 mg subcutaneously than at 2.5 mg. However, even at the lower doses used after restarting trials, there was a clear dose-response relationship to rapidly progressive OA and to progression to joint replacement. In addition, although these agents are efficacious, they may not provide a dramatic benefit over current OA therapy; in the earlier trials, even at the higher doses of 10 mg of tanezumab, the actual effect sizes[53] were not greatly superior to conventional OA treatments.[54] Nonetheless, on the basis of the positive phase 3 trial results, Pfizer has announced that it has submitted an application to the FDA for approval of tanezumab 2.5 mg for the treatment of knee OA (https://www.pfizer.com/news/press-release/press-release-detail/u_s_fda_accepts_regulatory_submission_for_tanezumab_a_potential_first_in_class_treatment_for_patients_with_chronic_pain_due_to_moderate_to_severe_osteoarthritis).

POPULAR AND HEAVILY MARKETED UNCONVENTIONAL STRATEGIES

As conventional treatments for OA pain have not fully relieved patients' pain, a large commercial market has developed that offers various biologically plausible approaches. This market is largely unregulated, but many of the approaches are marketed with promises of dramatic relief without surgery. Before considering individual treatments, it is essential to understand the role of the placebo effect in OA pain.

Contextual Effect

To fully appreciate the results of OA pain trials in general, it is essential to understand the role that the contextual effect plays in this disease. The contextual effect is the sum of all of the factors that comprise a response to a treatment except for the direct effect of that therapy itself. Thus, additional extraneous therapies, the natural history of the disease, and the social context of the patient may each contribute to the outcome. Importantly, this also includes the placebo effect, which is the benefit obtained from an inactive placebo agent. It has been known for years that OA pain is sensitive to placebos. Hence, in blinded placebo-controlled trials, the subjects receiving placebo routinely obtain clinically significant pain improvement. The magnitude of this improvement can be substantial, typically greater than a 40% reduction in pain.[55] Moreover, there is evidence that intra-articular placebo treatments may have significantly greater placebo effects than orally administered placebo.[56] The role that the placebo effect plays in OA therapeutics was evaluated systematically by Zou and colleagues, who reported that across 215 OA trials, approximately 75% of the pain reduction in the treatment groups was attributable to the placebo response.[57] Similar findings have been described when treatment options are limited to nonpharmacological approaches.[58] In light of the dramatic efficacy of placebos, the utility of novel OA therapies must be evaluated with clear reference to whether they are superior to the already high level of pain relief provided by placebos.

   The placebo effect is particularly important in understanding the popularity of some alternative modalities. For example, glucosamine and chondroitin sulfate have been popular dietary supplements for decades, with many OA patients deriving symptomatic relief. These have good safety profiles, assuming that they are manufactured using good manufacturing practice. However, there is compelling evidence that they do not provide substantial benefit beyond the placebo effect, although as previously noted, the placebo effect is potent in OA. There was great interest in these agents in the

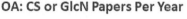

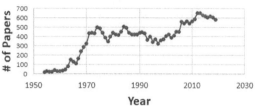

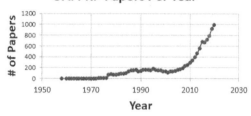

Fig. 1. The total number of publications related to glucosamine (GlcN) and chondroitin sulfate (CS) in OA, Top Panel, and to PRP in OA, as indexed by PubMed, by year. Top Panel: For GlcN/CS, there was great interest in the later years of the 20th century, which started to decline as large controlled studies failed to demonstrate substantial benefit. Interest in these agents recovered, however, as they remain in popular use, although it has been difficult to demonstrate clinically significant benefit beyond the contextual effects, as described in the text. Lower Panel: Interest in PRP for treating OA had an exponential increase, as measured by total PubMed-indexed publications, in the early 21st century, which appears to be coincident with the availability of devices that prepare the PRP in the United States, after initial clearance by the FDA.

late 20th century (**Fig. 1**, top panel), and early literature was enthusiastic; however, the studies suffered from high levels of design and publication bias. Subsequently, independently funded studies have consistently failed to demonstrate clinically significant benefit beyond placebo,[59,60] and these agents are not recommended by current OARSI or ACR guidelines.[12,13] Nonetheless, these agents remain widely used, and in light of the substantial placebo effect, they appear to provide substantial relief to many individuals.

ATTEMPTS AT DISEASE MODIFICATION

As noted previously, there are no treatments or strategies that have been shown to effectively retard the natural history of OA in people, despite several decades of investigation. Most of the modalities that have attracted attention as alternative approaches to OA pain were initiated as attempts to modify disease progression, especially through protection or repair of articular cartilage. Hence, most have underlying biological rationales that may well be plausible. However, whereas these modalities began as attempts to alter the structural progression or to repair cartilage, they are typically marketed as pain-palliating therapies.

Stem Cell Therapy

Adult articular cartilage is a nonreparative tissue, and once damaged, it tends to fibrillate and degenerate over time. When OA was considered to be merely a disease of degenerative cartilage, efforts were made to regenerate biomechanically functional cartilage. When it became clear that stem cells could be induced to differentiate along a chondrocytic lineage, there was hope that this might be a strategy to repair human cartilage, and stem cells have been an attractive target for OA therapy since the late 20th century. There are numerous ongoing efforts to engineer functional cartilage using stem cell technology, but the clinical use of stem cells today depends on the injection of free stem cells rather than on inserting engineered neocartilage into defective joints. The hope is that by injecting these cells into the synovial cavity, they will adhere to the joint surface and begin to synthesize cartilage-like matrix and anti-inflammatory mediators that will palliate pain. Normally, if a specific product were to be marketed for such an indication, it would require FDA approval and be required to demonstrate that it is both safe and effective. However, as these are clinical procedures and do not utilize standardized products, the intra-articular injection of stem cells is not regulated. Nonetheless, this has been studied in translational animal models. A recent systematic review of structural benefit and pain palliation of stem cell injections in animals, which assessed gross morphology, histologic and immunohistological analyses, radiography, and behavior analyses, found that any evidence to support benefit was of low quality.[61] Evidence of efficacy is equally scarce in people. A PubMed search using the keywords "osteoarthritis" and "stem cells" and "humans" yielded 1382 hits, although only 32 were controlled trials. In addition, there were 28 systematic reviews (pubmed.ncbi.nlm.nih.gov, searched 06/25/2020). Sources of the stem cells included autologous and allogenic adipose tissue, bone marrow, placenta, and peripheral blood. The systematic reviews generally reported that there was a positive response to pain with stem cell therapy, although there was heterogeneity and lack of reproducibility in the methodology, and no clear structural advantage.[62] Importantly, there is a consensus that current evidence does not support the use of intraarticular stem cells,[63] nor are they recommended by either the OARSI or ACR guidelines.[12,13] Notwithstanding the lack of compelling evidence, stem cell injections are widely used in people; in the United States, the number of clinics offering stem cell injections almost doubled between 2016 and 2018, to more than 700 nationwide.[64] This procedure is not typically covered by insurance and is cash only. The costs have been estimated as averaging more than $5000 per procedure, and patients surveyed afterward appear overwhelmingly satisfied with their results.[65] The discordance between objective evidence of benefit and satisfaction with treatment may be best explained by the extremely potent placebo effect in OA pain, especially when used with intra-articular injections.

Platelet-Rich Plasma

Platelet-rich plasma (PRP) is the name given to any preparation of autologous plasma whose platelet count is higher than that in the circulating blood (ie, it is enriched for platelets). This is typically prepared in a point-of-care process that involves centrifugation steps to separate plasma enriched with platelets. The resulting preparation is then injected intra-articularly in an attempt to palliate knee OA. Although marketing efforts frequently refer to this process as having FDA approval, in fact there is no approved indication for PRP; rather the devices that prepare the PRP are cleared by the FDA under a process known as 510(K) clearance, whereby the device itself is declared to be technically safe (ie, the resultant plasma product is not hazardous, and the performance has been shown to be technically similar to prior approved devices). In contrast to approval, which requires demonstration that the process is safe and effective, 510(K) clearance does not typically require demonstration of efficacy.[66] The FDA granted 510(K) clearance at least by 2011 for PRP processing,[67] and it is likely not a coincidence that interest in the literature had an exponential expansion at that time (see **Fig. 1**, lower panel). In addition to the absence of formal approval for the use of PRP in knee OA, there is no standardization regarding the volume of plasma to be injected, the degree of platelet enrichment, or the frequency of injections. Despite the variability in regimens, evidence of actual efficacy in OA remains sparse. As noted, it was originally developed as a strategy to modify disease progression. However, there is little evidence to suggest that it has important structural effects on articular pathology, nor is there apparently much effort to assess the structural benefit of PRP. A Clinicaltrials.gov search using the search terms "osteoarthritis" and "platelet rich plasma" revealed a listing of 107 relevant trials, of which only 6 had sought structural outcomes (https://clinicaltrials.gov/ct2/results?term=platelet+rich+plasma&cond=Osteoarthritis&draw=2&rank=104#rowId103, searched 9 July 2020). In addition to there being a paucity of data suggesting structural benefit, there are few data of actual efficacy of PRP beyond the anticipated placebo effect for knee OA. A PubMed search using search terms "osteoarthritis" and "humans" and "platelet rich plasma" and "clinical trials" revealed 54 studies (PubMed searched 9 July 2020), of which only 18 were actually controlled trials of PRP for OA, including 1 trial for hip OA. An additional 5 trials were systematic or narrative reviews. Most studies reported that PRP was safe and that it provided comparable pain and functional relief to comparators, such as hyaluronan injection or glucocorticoid injection, although there was no compelling evidence that it was a superior modality. Systematic reviews and meta-analyses have been performed, and generally have described high risk of bias and heterogeneity among the clinical trials.[68] Importantly, even meta-analyses whose authors tried to impute significant effect to PRP were unable to demonstrate such effect statistically and were left to conclude that there was a great deal of uncertainty.[69] This is especially relevant to clinicians who choose to recommend the therapy, as it is not typically covered by medical insurance and involves substantial out-of-pocket costs; recent surveys suggest that a single injection averages $714 and may be as much as $1390.[70]

It is important to appreciate that the published literature includes a variety of protocols, with the PRP preparations including platelet concentrations between twofold and eightfold blood levels, variable volumes, and with the frequency of treatment varying between once and multiple injections. As noted previously, there is inadequate evidence to conclude that any particular regimen is superior to others, or in fact superior to other comparators. Hence, the choice of frequency of injections and platelet preparation styles becomes largely one of personal preference and appears to be arbitrary.

Arthroscopy

It is noteworthy that arthroscopic lavage and debridement continue to be used for knee OA. There have been several controlled clinical trials that have failed to demonstrate benefit from this modality, beginning with a landmark study published in 2002.[71] Nonetheless, arthroscopy remains extremely common as treatment for knee OA,[72] despite its demonstrated lack of efficacy. Patients appear to be satisfied with the results, and this can likely be attributed to the impact of the placebo effect.

SUMMARY

Knee OA is a common painful disease, especially among middle-aged and elderly patients, and results in enormous societal morbidity and costs. There are no modalities that have been shown to alter the progression of the disease in people, and the primary goal of therapy at present is to relieve pain and to preserve function.

Notwithstanding enormous efforts over the past 50 years, OA pain remains inadequately controlled. Patient education and adjunctive measures are important, and exercise, physical therapy, and maintaining periarticular muscle strength relieve pain. Topical agents, especially NSAIDs, are effective and well tolerated; however, oral NSAIDs remain the mainstays of therapy, despite the attendant risks of chronic use. Neuroactive agents, such as duloxetine, are important for the non-nociceptive components of OA pain, and intra-articular therapies, including glucocorticoids and hyaluronans, have been used to provide short-term relief. OA pain is extraordinarily susceptible to the placebo effect, and the efficacy of novel therapeutics needs to be assessed through an appreciation of the placebo effect. Biological-based therapeutics are under development; anti-NGF antibody therapy is under FDA consideration. It has been shown to be effective for OA pain; however, the effect size is not as great as desired, and there are attendant risks. Various commercially successful and expensive modalities are in widespread use, although without clear data of their superiority to placebo. These include intra-articular stem cell injections and PRP. The next few years will see multiple new targets for OA pain, but a likely successful approach to disease modification is not yet defined.

CLINICS CARE POINTS

- The focus of knee OA management is on relieving pain and preserving function, as there are no pharmacologic or nonpharmacologic therapies that have been shown to delay progression of knee OA.

- NSAID therapy (including topical application) remains the cornerstone of knee OA management in appropriate patients. Acetaminophen may be useful for short-term pain control but is not effective for the management of chronic OA pain.

- The placebo effect is potent for OA pain, and most of the effect of all currently used OA therapies may be ascribed to this effect. Hence, this must be considered when choosing therapeutic strategies.

- There is a lack of evidence demonstrating efficacy above the placebo effect for intra-articular PRP or stem cell therapy, and such interventions involve costly out-of-pocket expenditures.

DISCLOSURE

J.A. Block: In the last 12 months, J.A. Block has received royalties for intellectual property (human chondrosarcoma cell lines) from Daiichi-Sankyo, Agios, and Omeros, and has received clinical trial funds from Novartis, Pfizer, Janssen, and TissueGene. He served as Chair of a DSMB for Discgenics and for the NIH/KAI Research Inc., and has consulted for Bioventus, GlaxoSmithKline, and Medivir. He receives compensation as editor in chief of *Osteoarthritis and Cartilage*. D. Cherny has no disclosures.

REFERENCES

1. Puig-Junoy J, Ruiz Zamora A. Socio-economic costs of osteoarthritis: a systematic review of cost-of-illness studies. Semin Arthritis Rheum 2015;44(5):531–41.
2. Zhao X, Shah D, Gandhi K, et al. Clinical, humanistic, and economic burden of osteoarthritis among noninstitutionalized adults in the United States. Osteoarthritis Cartilage 2019;27(11):1618–26.

3. Lawrence RC, Felson DT, Helmick CG, et al. Estimates of the prevalence of arthritis and other rheumatic conditions in the United States. Part II. Arthritis Rheum 2008;58(1):26–35.

4. Murphy L, Schwartz TA, Helmick CG, et al. . Lifetime risk of symptomatic knee osteoarthritis. Arthritis Rheum 2008;59(9):1207–13.

5. Castrejon I, Shakoor N, Chua JR, et al. Discordance of global assessment by patients and physicians is higher in osteoarthritis than in rheumatoid arthritis: a cross-sectional study from routine care. Rheumatol Int 2018;38(11):2137–45.

6. Chua JR, Jamal S, Riad M, et al. Disease burden in osteoarthritis is similar to that of rheumatoid arthritis at initial rheumatology visit and significantly greater six months later. Arthritis Rheumatol 2019;71(8):1276–84.

7. Pincus T, Castrejon I, Yazici Y, et al. Osteoarthritis is as severe as rheumatoid arthritis: evidence over 40 years according to the same measure in each disease. Clin Exp Rheumatol 2019;37 Suppl 120(5):7–17.

8. Loeser RF Jr. Aging and the etiopathogenesis and treatment of osteoarthritis. Rheum Dis Clin North Am 2000;26(3):547–67.

9. Hannan MT, Felson DT, Pincus T. Analysis of the discordance between radiographic changes and knee pain in osteoarthritis of the knee. J Rheumatol 2000;27(6):1513–7.

10. Block JA. Clinical features of osteoarthritis. In: Hochberg MGE, Silman A, Smolen J, et al, editors. Rheumatology, vol. 2, 7th edition. Elsevier; 2018. p. 1522–9.

11. Pincus T. Block JA. Pain and radiographic damage in osteoarthritis. BMJ 2009; 339:b2802.

12. Kolasinski SL, Neogi T, Hochberg MC, et al. 2019 American College of Rheumatology/Arthritis Foundation Guideline for the Management of Osteoarthritis of the Hand, Hip, and Knee. Arthritis Rheumatol 2020;72(2):220–33.

13. Bannuru RR, Osani MC, Vaysbrot EE, et al. . OARSI guidelines for the nonsurgical management of knee, hip, and polyarticular osteoarthritis. Osteoarthritis Cartilage 2019;27(11):1578–89.

14. Somers TJ, Wren AA, Shelby RA. The context of pain in arthritis: self-efficacy for managing pain and other symptoms. Curr Pain Headache Rep 2012;16(6):502–8.

15. Bliddal H, Leeds AR, Stigsgaard L, et al. Weight loss as treatment for knee osteoarthritis symptoms in obese patients: 1-year results from a randomised controlled trial. Ann Rheum Dis 2011;70(10):1798–803.

16. Messier SP, Resnik AE, Beavers DP, et al. Intentional weight loss in overweight and obese patients with knee osteoarthritis: is more better? Arthritis Care Res (Hoboken) 2018;70(11):1569–75.

17. Golightly YM, Allen KD, Caine DJ. A comprehensive review of the effectiveness of different exercise programs for patients with osteoarthritis. Phys Sportsmed 2012; 40(4):52–65.

18. Goh SL, Persson MSM, Stocks J, et al. Relative efficacy of different exercises for pain, function, performance and quality of life in knee and hip osteoarthritis: systematic review and network meta-analysis. Sports Med 2019;49(5):743–61.

19. Sugimoto D, Myer GD, Barber Foss KD, et al. Critical components of neuromuscular training to reduce ACL injury risk in female athletes: meta-regression analysis. Br J Sports Med 2016;50(20):1259–66.

20. Block JA, Shakoor N. Lower limb osteoarthritis: biomechanical alterations and implications for therapy. [Review]. Curr Opin Rheumatol 2010;22(5):544–50.

21. Simic M, Bennell K, Hunt M, et al. Contralateral cane use and knee joint load in people with medial knee osteoarthritis: the effect of varying body weight support. Osteoarthritis Cartilage 2011;19:1330–7.
22. Fregly BJ, D'Lima DD, Colwell CW Jr. Effective gait patterns for offloading the medial compartment of the knee. J Orthop Res 2009;27(8):1016–1021..
23. Van Ginckel A, Hinman RS, Wrigley TV, et al. Effect of cane use on bone marrow lesion volume in people with medial tibiofemoral knee osteoarthritis: randomized clinical trial. Osteoarthritis Cartilage 2019;27(9):1324–38.
24. Duivenvoorden T, Brouwer RW, van Raaij TM, et al. Braces and orthoses for treating osteoarthritis of the knee. Cochrane Database Syst Rev 2015;(3):CD004020.
25. Anand P, Bley K. Topical capsaicin for pain management: therapeutic potential and mechanisms of action of the new high-concentration capsaicin 8% patch. Br J Anaesth 2011;107(4):490–502.
26. Derry S, Wiffen PJ, Kalso EA, et al. Topical analgesics for acute and chronic pain in adults - an overview of Cochrane Reviews. Cochrane Database Syst Rev 2017;(5):CD008609.
27. Cameron M, Chrubasik S. Topical herbal therapies for treating osteoarthritis. Cochrane Database Syst Rev 2013;(5):CD010538.
28. Derry S, Conaghan P, Da Silva JA, et al. Topical NSAIDs for chronic musculoskeletal pain in adults. Cochrane Database Syst Rev 2016;(4):CD007400.
29. Bradley JD, Brandt KD, Katz BP, et al. Comparison of an antiinflammatory dose of ibuprofen, an analgesic dose of ibuprofen, and acetaminophen in the treatment of patients with osteoarthritis of the knee.[see comment]. N Engl J Med 1991; 325(2):87–91.
30. Case JP, Baliunas AJ, Block JA. Lack of efficacy of acetaminophen in treating symptomatic knee osteoarthritis: a randomized, double-blind, placebo-controlled comparison trial with diclofenac sodium. Arch Intern Med 2003;163(2):169–78.
31. Leopoldino AO, Machado GC, Ferreira PH, et al. Paracetamol versus placebo for knee and hip osteoarthritis. Cochrane Database Syst Rev 2019;(2):CD013273.
32. Schnitzer TJ, Hochberg MC, Marrero CE, et al. Efficacy and safety of naproxcinod in patients with osteoarthritis of the knee: a 53-week prospective randomized multicenter study. Semin Arthritis Rheum 2011;40(4):285–97.
33. Sheldon EA, Beaulieu A, Paster Z, et al. Long-term efficacy and safety of lumiracoxib 100 mg: an open-label extension of a 13-week randomized controlled trial in patients with primary osteoarthritis of the knee. Clin Exp Rheumatol 2008;26(4): 611–9.
34. Watson M, Brookes ST, Faulkner A, et al. Non-aspirin, non-steroidal anti-inflammatory drugs for treating osteoarthritis of the knee. Cochrane Database Syst Rev 2006;1
35. Woolf CJ. Capturing novel non-opioid pain targets. Biol Psychiatry 2020;87(1): 74–81.
36. Gao SH, Huo JB, Pan QM, et al. The short-term effect and safety of duloxetine in osteoarthritis: A systematic review and meta-analysis. Medicine 2019;98(44): e17541.
37. Noble M, Treadwell JR, Tregear SJ, et al. Long-term opioid management for chronic noncancer pain. Cochrane Database Syst Rev 2010;2010(1):CD006605.
38. da Costa BR, Nüesch E, Kasteler R, et al. Oral or transdermal opioids for osteoarthritis of the knee or hip. Cochrane Database Syst Rev 2014;(9):CD003115.
39. Lo-Ciganic WH, Floden L, Lee JK, et al. Analgesic use and risk of recurrent falls in participants with or at risk of knee osteoarthritis: data from the Osteoarthritis Initiative. Osteoarthritis Cartilage 2017;25(9):1390–8.

40. Cepeda MS, Camargo F, Zea C, et al. Tramadol for osteoarthritis. [Review] [71 refs]. Cochrane Database Syst Rev 2006;(3):CD005522.
41. Toupin April K, Bisaillon J, Welch V, et al. Tramadol for osteoarthritis. Cochrane Database Syst Rev 2019;(5):CD005522.
42. Jüni P, Hari R, Rutjes AW, et al. Intra-articular corticosteroid for knee osteoarthritis. Cochrane Database Syst Rev 2015;(10):CD005328.
43. McAlindon TE, LaValley MP, Harvey WF, et al. Effect of Intra-articular Triamcinolone vs Saline on Knee Cartilage Volume and Pain in Patients With Knee Osteoarthritis: A Randomized Clinical Trial. JAMA 2017;317(19):1967–75.
44. Conaghan PG, Hunter DJ, Cohen SB, et al. Effects of a single intra-articular injection of a microsphere formulation of triamcinolone acetonide on knee osteoarthritis pain: a double-blinded, randomized, placebo-controlled, multinational study. J Bone Joint Surg Am 2018;100(8):666–77.
45. Richardson C, Plaas A, Block JA. Intra-articular hyaluronan therapy for symptomatic knee osteoarthritis. Rheum Dis Clin North Am 2019;45(3):439–51.
46. Trojian TH, Concoff AL, Joy SM, et al. AMSSM scientific statement concerning viscosupplementation injections for knee osteoarthritis: importance for individual patient outcomes. Clin J Sport Med 2016;26(1):1–11.
47. Malfait AM, Miller RE, Block JA. Targeting neurotrophic factors: novel approaches to musculoskeletal pain. Pharmacol Ther 2020;211:107553.
48. Miller RE, Block JA, Malfait AM. What is new in pain modification in osteoarthritis? Rheumatology (Oxford) 2018;57(suppl_4):iv99–107.
49. Levi-Montalcini R, Hamburger V. Selective growth stimulating effects of mouse sarcoma on the sensory and sympathetic nervous system of the chick embryo. J Exp Zool 1951;116(2):321–61.
50. Lane NE, Schnitzer TJ, Birbara CA, et al. Tanezumab for the treatment of pain from osteoarthritis of the knee. N Engl J Med 2010;363(16):1521–31.
51. Schnitzer TJ, Easton R, Pang S, et al. Effect of tanezumab on joint pain, physical function, and patient global assessment of osteoarthritis among patients with osteoarthritis of the hip or knee: a randomized clinical trial. JAMA 2019;322(1):37–48.
52. Berenbaum F, Blanco FJ, Guermazi A, et al. . Subcutaneous tanezumab for osteoarthritis of the hip or knee: efficacy and safety results from a 24-week randomised phase III study with a 24-week follow-up period. Ann Rheum Dis 2020;79(6):800–10.
53. Schnitzer TJ, Marks JA. A systematic review of the efficacy and general safety of antibodies to NGF in the treatment of OA of the hip or knee. Osteoarthritis Cartilage 2015;23(Suppl 1):S8–17.
54. Block JA. Osteoarthritis: OA guidelines: improving care or merely codifying practice? Nat Rev Rheumatol 2014;10(6):324–6.
55. Doherty M, Dieppe P. The "placebo" response in osteoarthritis and its implications for clinical practice. Osteoarthritis Cartilage 2009;17(10):1255–62.
56. Bannuru RR, McAlindon TE, Sullivan MC, et al. Effectiveness and implications of alternative placebo treatments: a systematic review and network meta-analysis of osteoarthritis trials. Ann Intern Med 2015;163(5):365–72.
57. Zou K, Wong J, Abdullah N, et al. Examination of overall treatment effect and the proportion attributable to contextual effect in osteoarthritis: meta-analysis of randomised controlled trials. Ann Rheum Dis 2016;75(11):1964–70.
58. Chen AT, Shrestha S, Collins JE, et al. Estimating contextual effect in nonpharmacological therapies for pain in knee osteoarthritis: a systematic analytic review. Osteoarthritis Cartilage 2020;28(9):1154–69.

59. Liu X, Machado G, Eyles J, et al. Dietary supplements for treating osteoarthritis: a systematic review and meta-analysis. Br J Sports Med 2018;52(3):167–75.
60. Block JA, Oegema TR, Sandy JD, et al. The effects of oral glucosamine on joint health: is a change in research approach needed?. [Review] [84 refs]. Osteoarthritis Cartilage 2010;18(1):5–11.
61. Xing D, Kwong J, Yang Z, et al. Intra-articular injection of mesenchymal stem cells in treating knee osteoarthritis: a systematic review of animal studies. Osteoarthritis Cartilage 2018;26(4):445–61.
62. Jevotovsky DS, Alfonso AR, Einhorn TA, et al. Osteoarthritis and stem cell therapy in humans: a systematic review. Osteoarthritis Cartilage 2018;26(6):711–29.
63. Kim SH, Ha CW, Park YB, et al. Intra-articular injection of mesenchymal stem cells for clinical outcomes and cartilage repair in osteoarthritis of the knee: a meta-analysis of randomized controlled trials. Arch Orthop Trauma Surg 2019;139(7): 971–80.
64. Knoepfler PS, Turner LG. The FDA and the US direct-to-consumer marketplace for stem cell interventions: a temporal analysis. Regen Med 2018;13(1):19–27.
65. Piuzzi NS, Ng M, Chughtai M, et al. The stem-cell market for the treatment of knee osteoarthritis: a patient perspective. J Knee Surg 2018;31(6):551–6.
66. Beitzel K, Allen D, Apostolakos J, et al. US definitions, current use, and FDA stance on use of platelet-rich plasma in sports medicine. J Knee Surg 2015; 28(1):29–34.
67. Yuan XJ, Gellhorn AC. Platelet rich plasma. In: Cooper G, Herrera J, Kirkbride J, et al, editors. Regenerative medicine for spine and joint pain. Cham: Springer International Publishing; 2020. p. 55–86.
68. Laudy AB, Bakker EW, Rekers M, et al. Efficacy of platelet-rich plasma injections in osteoarthritis of the knee: a systematic review and meta-analysis. Br J Sports Med 2015;49(10):657–72.
69. Vannabouathong C, Bhandari M, Bedi A, et al. Nonoperative treatments for knee osteoarthritis: an evaluation of treatment characteristics and the intra-articular placebo effect: a systematic review. JBJS Rev 2018;6(7):e5.
70. Piuzzi NS, Ng M, Kantor A, et al. What is the price and claimed efficacy of platelet-rich plasma injections for the treatment of knee osteoarthritis in the United States? J Knee Surg 2019;32(9):879–85.
71. Moseley JB, O'Malley K, Petersen NJ, et al. A controlled trial of arthroscopic surgery for osteoarthritis of the knee. N Engl J Med 2002;347(2):81–8.
72. Adelani MA, Harris AHS, Bowe TR, et al. Arthroscopy for knee osteoarthritis has not decreased after a clinical trial. Clin Orthop Relat Res 2016;474(2):489–94.

Antinuclear Antibody Testing for the Diagnosis of Systemic Lupus Erythematosus

Rand A. Nashi, MD[a], Robert H. Shmerling, MD[a,b,c],*

KEYWORDS

- Antinuclear antibody (ANA) • SLE • Sensitivity • Specificity • Predictive value
- Diagnosis

KEY POINTS

- Systemic lupus erythematosus (SLE) is a systemic autoimmune inflammatory condition that may involve multiple organ systems.
- Although the antinuclear antibody (ANA) test is positive in nearly every case of SLE, it is not specific for this disease and, therefore, must be interpreted in the appropriate clinical context.
- Key features that may warrant ANA testing include unexplained multisystem inflammatory disease, symmetric joint pain with inflammatory features, photosensitive rash, and cytopenias.
- In select cases, ANA staining patterns and more specific autoantibody testing may be helpful in suggesting a diagnosis of suspected SLE or another ANA-associated disease.
- For patients with nonspecific symptoms, such as malaise and fatigue (who have a low likelihood of SLE or a related disease), ANA testing is of limited value.

INTRODUCTION

Systemic lupus erythematosus (SLE) is a systemic autoimmune inflammatory condition that may cause inflammation and damage in multiple organ systems and is associated with significant morbidity and premature death. It affects people of all ethnicities and geographic locations. Estimates suggest a female prevalence that is 10 times higher than among men and, within the United States, groups at elevated risk include African American and Hispanics/Latinx communities.[1] In addition to its direct impact on multiple organ systems, SLE is associated with morbidity related

This article originally appeared in the Medical Clinics of North America, Volume 105, Issue 2, March 2021.

[a] Division of Rheumatology, Beth Israel Deaconess Medical Center, 110 Francis Street, Suite 4B, Boston, MA 02215, USA; [b] Harvard Health Publications, Harvard Medical School, Boston, MA, USA; [c] Harvard Medical School, Boston, MA, USA

* Corresponding author. 110 Francis Street, Suite 4B, Boston, MA 02215.

E-mail address: rshmerli@bidmc.harvard.edu

to cardiovascular disease and malignancy,[2] presumably due to a chronically height-ened inflammatory state.

SLE may be difficult to diagnose due to the diversity of presenting symptoms and signs and because its symptoms are common and nonspecific. Although symptoms, such as arthritis and the classic malar rash, may be readily recognized, other presen-tations, such as hemolytic anemia, seizures, or psychosis, alone or even in combina-tion, may be attributed to other causes or conditions. Furthermore, the challenge of diagnosis is compounded by the lack of a single gold standard test. Although a pos-itive antinuclear antibody (ANA) test is a clue, it must be considered within the context of other clinical features, including details of the history, physical examination, and other test results.

The pathophysiology of SLE is incompletely understood. Several factors have been linked to its development and expression, including genetic, hormonal, and environ-mental influences.[3] Studies examining monozygotic twins have found SLE concor-dance of 24% to 57%.[4,5] But genetics alone do not fully explain disease manifestations. Other important pathogenetic factors may include exposure to hor-mones, such as estrogen (which is believed to be pathogenic in murine models of SLE) and exposure to ultraviolet light. Impaired clearance of apoptotic cellular debris and a dysregulated immune response to self-antigens may be important in triggering SLE or flares of the disease.[6] These processes may act in synergy to impair the host's self-tolerance and immune regulation, leading to the development of autoantibodies and immune complex deposition, the primary drivers of organ damage and clinical manifestations.

THE CLINICAL USEFULNESS OF ANTINUCLEAR ANTIBODY TESTING

ANAs are a collection of autoantibodies that target proteins within the nucleus of the cell. A positive result can signify breakdown of self-tolerance and herald the onset of autoimmune disease, such as SLE. A patient's ANA may be positive, however, in a va-riety of other settings and even may be present in healthy individuals. As a result, the usefulness of any individual's ANA test result is highly dependent on that individual's specific clinical presentation and pretest probability of SLE or other ANA-associated disease.

The ANA typically is reported as a titer, a quantitative measure of the amount of anti-body, expressed as the number of dilutions a sample can undergo and still demon-strate detectable antibody. An ANA of 1:40, for example, is a low titer found in many people without autoimmune disease and, in some laboratories, is considered negative. The most recent classification criteria from for SLE from the European League Against Rheumatism (EULAR) and the American College of Rheumatology (ACR)[7] require a titer of at least 1:80 for consideration of the diagnosis. In general, the higher the ANA titer, the more likely the result is an indication of autoimmunity,[8] but the ANA titer is not an accurate reflection of disease activity.

A range of sensitivities and specificities for ANA testing have been reported; this is not surprising because the types of patients tested and methodologies used for testing vary. Indirect immunofluorescence using human epithelial type 2 (HEp-2) cell lines and solid-phase testing techniques (including enzyme immunoassays and multi-plex bead assays) currently are the most common ways to assess the presence of an ANA; the former is the most widely used and is recommended by the ACR[9] as the gold standard methodology. Solid-phase immunoassays may be less expensive to perform, easier to standardize, more efficient, and less expensive to perform; howev-er, lower sensitivity has been a limiting factor.

According to a recent meta-regression analysis of ANA tests (96% of which used indirect immunofluorescence with HEp-2 cell substrate),[10] a positive ANA at a titer of 1:80 had sensitivity of 98% and specificity of 75%. Given the high sensitivity of the ANA for SLE, a negative ANA is a powerful argument against the diagnosis. The modest specificity means, however, that unless testing is highly selective (ie, limited to settings of high pretest probability), false-positive results are common; this represents a significant limitation of the test.[11]

As a diagnostic test, the ANA test can be useful in suggesting the diagnosis of SLE but other diseases, including nonrheumatologic conditions, also are associated with a positive ANA. In addition to SLE, rheumatic diseases in which a positive ANA often is found include

- Systemic sclerosis (scleroderma)
- Sjögren syndrome
- Rheumatoid arthritis
- Dermatomyositis and polymyositis
- Drug-induced lupus

Nonrheumatologic diseases associated with a positive ANA include autoimmune thyroid disease (such as Hashimoto thyroiditis), autoimmune hepatitis, and primary biliary cholangitis. In addition, many infections and malignancies are associated with immune dysregulation and autoantibody formation that includes ANAs that may be present in high titers.[12,13]

As indicated by its limited specificity, ANAs often are positive in people without a clinically relevant disease; 25% or more of the population are ANA-positive even without a rheumatic disease or other ANA-associated condition. The prevalence of positive ANAs in the population may be rising in the United States,[14] although the clinical importance of this is unclear. A higher incidence of false-positive results may be found in individuals who are aged[15] or have a family member with a positive ANA or autoimmune disease.

For these reasons, a single ANA result does not have a single interpretation: a low-titer ANA in a patient without a strong clinical suggestion of SLE or other ANA-associated disease usually is of little clinical significance; however, that same result in a patient with a malar rash, inflammatory arthralgia, and hematuria may reflect the presence of a systemic rheumatic disease, such as SLE. The value of detecting a positive ANA in a patient with nonspecific symptoms (such as malaise, fatigue, and generalized pain) is low, particularly if more specific symptoms are absent and other laboratory studies, such as the complete blood cell count, renal function, and urinalysis, are normal.

ANTINUCLEAR ANTIBODY STAINING PATTERNS

ANAs typically are reported with a pattern of fluorescent staining, which can be a clue regarding the underlying antigen specificity:

- A homogenous staining pattern may reflect antibodies directed against histone proteins and DNA
- A speckled staining pattern may be due to antibodies against U1-ribonucleoprotein (RNP), Smith (Sm), and Ro and La antigens
- A nucleolar pattern often signifies antibodies against RNA polymerase
- A peripheral, or rim, staining pattern suggests the presence of anti–double-stranded (anti-ds) DNA antibodies

- A centromeric pattern typically is found in patients with CREST syndrome (discussed later)

Because certain antigen specificities are highly associated with particular diseases (eg, anti-Sm and anti-dsDNA antibodies are highly specific for SLE), these staining patterns can be clinically useful.[16] The interpretation and reporting of ANA patterns, however, may be operator-dependent and subject to interobserver variability. In addition, the correlation between staining pattern and specific diseases is not particularly strong.

TESTING FOR ANTIBODIES DIRECTED AGAINST SPECIFIC AUTOANTIGENS

ANAs may be positive due to antibodies directed against several autoantigens (often called extractable nuclear antibodies). Among the most common and clinically useful include

- Anti-dsDNA and anti-Sm antibodies—these are highly specific for SLE. In addition, anti-dsDNA antibodies may correlate with SLE disease activity, especially among those with nephritis.
- Anti-RNP antibodies are associated with mixed connective tissue disease and SLE. A positive anti-RNP antibody is not enough, however, to establish a diagnosis of either disease.
- Anti-Ro (anti-SSA) and anti-La (anti-SSB) antibodies are associated with primary Sjögren syndrome and SLE; in addition, anti-Ro antibodies are strongly linked to the development of neonatal lupus.
- Antihistone antibodies are present in approximately half of patients with SLE but nearly always are present in drug-induced lupus
- Anti–Scl-70 (anti-topoisomerase 3) and anti-RNA polymerase antibodies are highly specific for scleroderma.
- Anticentromere antibodies are strongly associated with the limited form of systemic sclerosis, or CREST syndrome (manifest by calcinosis, Raynaud phenomenon, esophageal dysmotility, sclerodactyly, and telangiectasia); they occasionally are present in patients with SLE.

As diagnostic tests, these antibodies are variably sensitive but their clinical value lies in their high specificity (**Table 1**). Testing for these more specific autoantibodies is not recommended routinely for patients who are ANA-negative or whose ANA status is unknown, especially in the setting of low pretest probability of disease.[17]

Table 1
Specific antinuclear antibodies, associated diseases, sensitivity, and specificity

Specific Antinuclear Antibody	Associated Disease	Sensitivity (%)	Specificity (%)
Anti-Sm	SLE	40[24]	98.6[24]
Anti-dsDNA	SLE	90[25]	96[25]
Anti-SSA (anti-Ro)	Primary Sjögren syndrome	49[26]	87.5[26]
Anti-SSB (anti-Lo)	Primary Sjögren syndrome	29[26]	95[26]
Anti-RNP	Mixed connective tissue disease	100[27]	84–100[28]
Anti–Scl-70	Systemic sclerosis (scleroderma)	28[29]	100[29]
Anticentromere	Limited scleroderma	33[30]	99.9[30]

HOW IS SYSTEMIC LUPUS ERYTHEMATOSUS DIAGNOSED?

A diagnosis of SLE requires a compelling combination of symptoms, physical examination findings, and laboratory and/or pathologic studies. Ultimately, clinical acumen and judgment are required to integrate the various features of the illness: asking the right questions, eliciting compatible physical findings, and interpreting the results of selected tests are essential. A young woman with diffuse aching and morning stiffness with a low-titer positive ANA could have fibromyalgia, SLE, a self-limited viral syndrome, or several other conditions. But, if she also has a family history of SLE, unexplained fever, and a photosensitive rash, the suspicion of SLE should rise much higher. And if these same symptoms were present in someone taking infliximab or procainamide, the possibility of drug-induced lupus would be appropriate. Thus, interpreting an ANA result requires an assessment of pretest probability, a recognition of its sensitivity and specificity, and an actual or estimated calculation of positive and negative predictive values.

The various iterations and revisions of lupus classification criteria can provide useful guidance for the evaluation of possible SLE. They include manifestations that are relatively common and, in cases of the 2019 EULAR/ACR classification criteria for SLE,[7] they provide a sense of how various manifestations of disease should be weighed (**Table 2**). For example, a renal biopsy demonstrating pathologic evidence of lupus nephritis is far more suggestive of the diagnosis than the (much less specific) finding of fever.

But, there is a reason the classification criteria are not called diagnostic criteria—a patient can have SLE without meeting these criteria or not have SLE even though meeting the criteria. These criteria are intended to standardize studies of the disease, not to be a tool to allow a clinician to establish or rule out the diagnosis in an individual patient.

Some aspects of the 2019 classification criteria for SLE[7] deserve particular emphasis:

- As discussed previously, a patient must have an ANA of at least 1:80 using a HEp-2 immunofluorescence assay (or an equivalent positive test).
- Criteria include 10 clinical or immunologic domains with 1 or more manifestations in each; only the highest scoring item within a domain can be counted (so a patient with discoid lupus and oral ulcers only gets credit for discoid lupus); each criterion has specific definitions (eg, fever must be >38.3°C and leukopenia is <4000 cells/mm^3).
- The 7 clinical domains are constitutional, hematologic, neuropsychiatric, mucocutaneous, serosal, musculoskeletal, and renal.
- The 3 immunology domains are antiphospholipid antibodies, complement proteins, and SLE-specific antibodies (anti-dsDNA or anti-Sm).
- A criterion should not be counted if there is a more likely explanation for it than SLE,
- Even with a positive ANA of at least 1:80 and at least 10 points, 1 or more clinical criteria must be met.
- Criteria do not have to be present at the same time,

Because a diagnosis of SLE has immediate as well as long-term implications with potential for a poor prognosis, a strong suspicion of SLE should prompt timely referral to a rheumatologist. The ANA is an important part of the evaluation but it is only 1 part of the diagnostic process. For nonrheumatologists, it probably is more important to decide whether to refer the patient based on clinical grounds to a rheumatologist and to determine how urgent that consultation should be than it is to decide whether an ANA should be requested.

Table 2
European League against Rheumatism/American College of Rheumatology classification criteria for systemic lupus erythematosus

Clinical Domains and Criteria	Weight (Points)
Constitutional	
Fever	2
Hematologic	
Leukopenia	3
Thrombocytopenia	4
Autoimmune hemolysis	4
Neuropsychiatric	
Delirium	2
Psychosis	3
Seizure	5
Mucocutaneous	
Nonscarring alopecia	2
Oral ulcers	2
Subacute cutaneous or discoid lupus	4
Acute cutaneous lupus	6
Serosal	
Pleural or pericardial effusion	5
Acute pericarditis	6
Musculoskeletal	
Joint involvement	6
Renal	
Proteinuria >0.5 g per 24 h	4
Renal biopsy class II or V lupus nephritis	8
Renal biopsy class III or IV lupus nephritis	10
Immunologic Domains and Criteria	**Weight (Points)**
Antiphospholipid antibodies	
Anticardiolipin antibodies OR anti–beta-2 glycoprotein 1 antibodies OR lupus anticoagulant	2
Complement proteins	
Low C3 OR low C4	3
Low C3 AND low C4	4
SLE-specific antibodies	
Anti-dsDNA OR anti-Sm antibodies	6

See text for details.
Adapted from Aringer M, Costenbader K, Daikh D, et al. 2019 European League Against Rheumatism/American College of Rheumatology classification criteria for systemic lupus erythematosus. Arthritis & Rheumatology 2019;71(9):1409; with permission.

WHEN IS IT APPROPRIATE TO ORDER AN ANTINUCLEAR ANTIBODY TEST?

Several studies have appropriately decried the problem of overtesting, over-reliance on test results, and/or the costs they incur.[18–20] There is little consensus, however, on the specific clinical scenarios for which it is appropriate to order an ANA. This is understandable: clinicians want to avoid delaying a diagnosis as important as SLE, the disease has protean manifestations, so testing may seem easy to justify, and the nonspecific nature of the presentation (eg, fatigue and anemia) makes casting a wide net a tempting approach. For patients with multiple, nonspecific symptoms, it can be a challenge to decide whether or not to request ANA testing.

In 2002, the ACR Ad Hoc Committee on Immunologic Testing Guidelines published a review of conditions in which ANA testing might be particularly useful.[21] It recommended ANA testing for a limited number of conditions, including a suspicion of SLE, systemic sclerosis, mixed connective tissue disease, or drug-induced lupus and stratifying risk of uveitis in patients with juvenile idiopathic arthritis. These guidelines did not specify which symptoms, signs, or other test results should make a clinician suspect SLE or other condition that would prompt ANA testing.

Although the presentation of SLE can vary widely, some clinical manifestations are more suggestive than others (as reflected by their weighting in the latest classification criteria[7]). The clinical setting and demographics of the patient matter: other (non-SLE) explanations must be considered and suggestive signs or symptoms are more likely to reflect SLE if they occur in a woman of childbearing age.

Here are some specific presentations that individually or in combination may warrant a high suspicion of SLE:

- Inflammatory polyarthralgia (including prolonged morning stiffness) or polyarthritis in a rheumatoid distribution (including metacarpophalangeal, proximal interphalangeal, and wrist joints)
- Persistent photosensitive rash (including a malar rash that spares the nasolabial fold), discoid lupus, and subacute or acute cutaneous lupus. These should be distinguished from more evanescent sun or heat triggered flushing.
- Hemolytic anemia or idiopathic thrombocytopenic purpura
- Unexplained and recurrent seizures or serositis
- Unexplained nephrotic syndrome or glomerulonephritis
- Multisystem inflammatory disease that otherwise is unexplained and includes features of the classification criteria[7]

Although the list of clinical presentations of SLE is long, the list of presentations in which SLE is unlikely is even longer. For example, individuals whose dominant symptoms are chronic low back pain, noninflammatory knee pain, or distal interphalangeal bony enlargement are unlikely to derive benefit from ANA testing. In such settings, a negative result is unlikely to add useful diagnostic information whereas a positive result likely is difficult to interpret and may lead to additional and unnecessary testing, referral, and treatment. Similarly, repeat ANA testing commonly is performed but rarely helpful.[20]

A major limitation of algorithms designed to guide clinicians through a rational sequence of diagnostic evaluation for suspected SLE is that the entry criterion is "suspicion of SLE."[22,23] Without providing details of why that diagnosis would be in play, it is unclear how useful such approaches may be.

SUMMARY

ANA testing clearly is an important part of the evaluation of a patient with possible SLE. It is important, however, to understand the strengths and weaknesses of the test and to interpret the results in the context of the specific clinical scenario that lead to testing in the first place. ANAs are present in nearly everyone with SLE but also may be present in other rheumatic disease, autoimmune thyroid disease, and liver disease and in many healthy individuals. Ideally, an ANA should be ordered only when there is at least a moderate clinical suspicion of SLE (or other ANA-associated disease) and when the results are likely to advance diagnostic confidence. Considering the protean manifestations of SLE and the innumerable permutations of their presentation, it is unlikely that counting up criteria or running clinical algorithms can do more than provide general guidance—the final determination relies on the expertise of the evaluating clinician.

CLINICS CARE POINTS

- Although ANA testing is an important part of the evaluation of a patient with possible SLE, a positive ANA is not specific for SLE because it may be associated with a variety of rheumatic and nonrheumatic diseases.

- Because of its high sensitivity in SLE, a negative ANA is a strong argument against the diagnosis.

- To optimize clinical utility, the ANA should be ordered when there is a significant clinical suspicion of an ANA-associated disease and the results help rule in or rule out that condition.

- Recent classification criteria for SLE require a positive ANA at a titer of at least 1:80, emphasizing both the importance of a positive ANA in the diagnosis and the uncertain relevance of a minimally positive result.

- Repeated ANA testing rarely is helpful.

- If there is enough concern about possible SLE (or other ANA-associated rheumatic disease) to request ANA testing, it generally is advisable also to order a complete blood cell count with differential, serum creatinine, and urinalysis.

DISCLOSURE

The authors have no financial conflicts to disclose.

REFERENCES

1. Stojan G, Petri M. Epidemiology of systemic lupus erythematosus: an update. Curr Opin Rheumatol 2018;30:144–50.
2. Ippolito A, Petri M. An update on mortality in systemic lupus erythematosus. Clin Exp Rheumatol 2008;26:S72.
3. Tsokos GC. Autoimmunity and organ damage in systemic lupus erythematosus. Nat Immunol 2020;21:605–14.
4. Block SR, Winfield JB, Lockshin MD, et al. Studies of twins with systemic lupus erythematosus. A review of the literature and presentation of 12 additional sets. Am J Med 1975;59:533–52.
5. Deapen D, Escalante A, Weinrib L, et al. A revised estimate of twin concordance in systemic lupus erythematosus. Arthritis Rheum 1992;35:311–8.
6. Yang F, He Y, Zhai Z, et al. Programmed Cell Death Pathways in the Pathogenesis of Systemic Lupus Erythematosus. J Immunol Res 2019;2019:3638562.
7. Aringer M, Costenbader K, Daikh D, et al. 2019 European League Against Rheumatism/American College of Rheumatology classification criteria for systemic lupus erythematosus. Arthritis Rheumatol 2019;71:1400–12.
8. Satoh M, Vázquez-Del Mercado M, Chan EK. Clinical interpretation of antinuclear antibody tests in systemic rheumatic diseases. Mod Rheumatol 2009;19:219–28.

9. American College of Rheumatology Position Statement, Methodology of Testing for Antinuclear Antibodies. 2009. Available at: https://www.rheumatology.org/Portals/0/Files/Methodology%20of%20Testing%20Antinuclear%20Antibodies%20Position%20Statement.pdf. Accessed July 12, 2020.

10. Leuchten N, Hoyer A, Brinks R, et al. Performance of Antinuclear Antibodies for Classifying Systemic Lupus Erythematosus: A Systematic Literature Review and Meta-Regression of Diagnostic Data. Arthritis Care Res (Hoboken) 2018; 70:428–38.

11. Slater CA, Davis RB, Shmerling RH. Antinuclear antibody testing. A study of clinical utility. Arch Intern Med 1996;156:1421–5.

12. Im JH, Chung M-H, Park YK, et al. Antinuclear antibodies in infectious diseases. Infect Dis 2020;52:177–85.

13. Solans-Laqué R, Pérez-Bocanegra C, Salud-Salvia A, et al. Clinical significance of antinuclear antibodies in malignant diseases: association with rheumatic and connective tissue paraneoplastic syndromes. Lupus 2004;13:159–64.

14. Dinse GE, Parks CG, Weinberg CR, et al. Increasing Prevalence of Antinuclear Antibodies in the United States. Arthritis Rheumatol 2020;72:1026–35.

15. Nilsson BO, Skogh T, Ernerudh J, et al. Antinuclear antibodies in the oldest-old women and men. J Autoimmun 2006;27:281–8.

16. Mariz HA, Sato EI, Barbosa SH, et al. Pattern on the antinuclear antibody–HEp-2 test is a critical parameter for discriminating antinuclear antibody–positive healthy individuals and patients with autoimmune rheumatic diseases. Arthritis Rheum 2011;63:191–200.

17. Choosing Wisely - American College of Rheumatology 2013. Available at: https://www.choosingwisely.org/clinician-lists/american-college-rheumatology-ana-sub-serologies-without-positive-ana-and-clinical-suspicion/?highlight=antinuclear%20antibody. Accessed July 19, 2020.

18. Mohammed AS, Boddu P, Mael D, et al. Inappropriate use of commercial Antinuclear Antibody Testing in a community-based US hospital: a retrospective study. J Community Hosp Intern Med Perspect 2016;6:32031.

19. Man A, Shojania K, Phoon C, et al. An evaluation of autoimmune antibody testing patterns in a Canadian health region and an evaluation of a laboratory algorithm aimed at reducing unnecessary testing. Clin Rheumatol 2013;32:601–8.

20. Yeo A, Ong J, Connelly K, et al. ANA-lysis: Utility of Repeated Antinuclear Antibody Testing in a Single Center [abstract]. Arthritis Rheumatol 2019;71(suppl 10). Available at: https://acrabstracts.org/abstract/ana-lysis-utility-of-repeated-antinuclear-antibody-testing-in-a-single-center/. Accessed October 20, 2020.

21. Solomon DH, Kavanaugh AJ, Schur PH. Evidence-based guidelines for the use of immunologic tests: Antinuclear antibody testing. Arthritis Rheum 2002;47:434–44.

22. Lam NC, Ghetu MV, Bieniek ML. Systemic lupus erythematosus: primary care approach to diagnosis and management. Am Fam Physician 2016;94:284–94.

23. Chen L, Welsh KJ, Chang B, et al. Algorithmic approach with clinical pathology consultation improves access to specialty care for patients with systemic lupus erythematosus. Am J Clin Pathol 2016;146:312–8.

24. Pan LT, Tin SK, Boey ML, et al. The sensitivity and specificity of autoantibodies to the Sm antigen in the diagnosis of systemic lupus erythematosus. Ann Acad Med Singapore 1998;27:21–3.

25. Wichainun R, Kasitanon N, Wangkaew S, et al. Sensitivity and specificity of ANA and anti-dsDNA in the diagnosis of systemic lupus erythematosus: a comparison using control sera obtained from healthy individuals and patients with multiple medical problems. Asian Pac J Allergy Immunol 2013;31:292.

26. Wei P, Li C, Qiang L, et al. Role of salivary anti-SSA/B antibodies for diagnosing primary Sjögren's syndrome. Med Oral Patol Oral Cir Bucal 2015;20:e156–60.

27. Dima A, Jurcut C, Baicus C. The impact of anti-U1-RNP positivity: systemic lupus erythematosus versus mixed connective tissue disease. Rheumatol Int 2018;38: 1169–78.

28. Benito-Garcia E, Schur PH, Lahita R, et al. Guidelines for immunologic laboratory testing in the rheumatic diseases: Anti-Sm and anti-RNP antibody tests. Arthritis Rheum 2004;51:1030–44.

29. Birtane M, Yavuz S, Taştekin N. Laboratory evaluation in rheumatic diseases. World J Methodol 2017;7:1–8.

30. Ho KT, Reveille JD. The clinical relevance of autoantibodies in scleroderma. Arthritis Res Ther 2003;5:80–93.

Printed and bound by CPI Group (UK) Ltd, Croydon, CR0 4YY

08/05/2025

01864716-0001